Second Edition

ACLS for EMTs

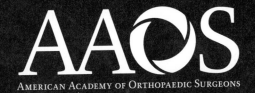

AMERICAN ACADEMY OF ORTHOPAEDIC SURGEONS

Author:
Mike Smith, BS, MICP

Program Chair, Lead Instructor,
Emergency Medical and Health Services

Tacoma Community College
Tacoma, Washington

Series Editor:

Andrew N. Pollak, MD, FAAOS

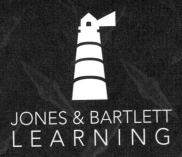

JONES & BARTLETT
LEARNING

World Headquarters
Jones & Bartlett Learning
5 Wall Street
Burlington, MA 01803
978-443-5000
info@jblearning.com
www.jblearning.com

Jones & Bartlett Learning books and products are available through most bookstores and online booksellers. To contact Jones & Bartlett Learning directly, call 800-832-0034, fax 978-443-8000, or visit our website, www.jblearning.com.

Substantial discounts on bulk quantities of Jones & Bartlett Learning publications are available to corporations, professional associations, and other qualified organizations. For details and specific discount information, contact the special sales department at Jones & Bartlett Learning via the above contact information or send an email to specialsales@jblearning.com.

Production Credits
Chief Executive Officer: Ty Field
President: James Homer
SVP, Editor-in-Chief: Michael Johnson
SVP, Chief Marketing Officer: Alison M. Pendergast
Executive Publisher: Kimberly Brophy
Executive Acquisitions Editor—EMS: Christine Emerton
Editor: Alison Lozeau
Production Manager: Jenny L. Corriveau
Production Editor: Marcia Murray
Vice President of Sales, Public Safety Group: Matthew Maniscalco
Director of Sales, Public Safety Group: Patricia Einstein
Director of Marketing: Alisha Weisman
VP, Manufacturing and Inventory Control: Therese Connell
Composition: diacriTech
Cover Design: Scott Moden
Rights & Photo Research Assistant: Gina Licata
Cover Image: © Stockbroker/MBI/Alamy Images
Printing and Binding: Courier Companies
Cover Printing: Courier Companies

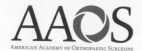

Library of Congress Cataloging-in-Publication Data Not Available at Time of Printing

6048

Printed in the United States of America
16 15 14 13 12   10 9 8 7 6 5 4 3 2 1

CONTENTS

CONTRIBUTORS

Jones & Bartlett Learning and the American Academy of Orthopaedic Surgeons would like to thank the following authors for their significant contributions to the text:

Rommie L. Duckworth, LP
Founder, Program Coordinator
New England Center for Rescue & Emergency
    Medicine, LLC
Sherman, Connecticut

Christopher Touzeau, MS, NREMT-P, RN
Maryland Fire and Rescue Institute
University of Maryland
Master Firefighter Paramedic
Montgomery County Fire and Rescue Service
Rockville, Maryland

ACKNOWLEDGMENTS

The American Academy of Orthopaedic Surgeons, the authors, and Jones & Bartlett Learning wish to thank the reviewers who were involved in the development of this resource:

Erik Bergsten, EMT Instructor
Law and Public Safety Institute – EMS Academy
Ramsey, New Jersey

Rob Bernini, EMT-P, CCEMT-P
Harrisburg Area Community College
Harrisburg, Pennsylvania

Harvey Conner, AS, NREMT-P
EMS Program
Oklahoma City Community College
Midwest City, Oklahoma

Heidi P. Cordi, MD, MPH, MS, EMTP, FACEP
The New York Presbyterian Hospital
Cordi Consultants, Inc.
Elmsford, New York

Clyde Deschamp, PhD, NREMT-P
University of Mississippi Medical Center
Jackson, Mississippi

Bob Elling, MPA, EMT-P
Hudson Valley Community College Paramedic
  Program
Troy, New York

Randy L. Fugate, NREMTP, CCEMTP, PNCCT
NC Level II Paramedic Instructor/Coordinator
Asheville–Buncombe Technical Community
  College
Mission Health System Regional Transport
  Services
Asheville, North Carolina

Marla A. Garza, NREMT-P
UTHSCSA
San Antonio, Texas

Robert M. Hawkes, MSPA, NREMT-P, PA-C
NOVA Southeastern University
Fort Myers, Florida

Mary Hewett, BS-EMS, NREMTP
BLS/ILS/Rural Programs Director
University of New Mexico
School of Medicine
EMS Academy
Albuquerque, New Mexico

Rick Hilinski, BA, EMT-P
Community College of Allegheny County
Pittsburgh, Pennsylvania

Roxane Horowitz, RN, BSN, NREMT, EMT-I
Education Manager/Program Coordinator
MONOC-New Jersey's Hospital Service Corp
Wall, New Jersey

Deb Kaye, BS, NREMT
EMT/First Responder Training Program
  Coordinator
Dakota County Technical College
Rosemount, Minnesota
EMT
Sunburg Ambulance and Lakes Area Rural
  Responders
Sunburg, Minnesota

Anton Preisinger
Lake Forest Park, Washington

ACKNOWLEDGMENTS

Scott Tomek, MA, Paramedic
Faculty
Century College Paramedic Program
White Bear Lake, Minnesota
Manager
Quality Improvement, Safety, & Risk
  Management
Allina Health EMS
St. Paul, Minnesota

David A. Young, BS, NREMT-P
Coordinator/Instructor EMS Programs
Western Piedmont Community College
Morganton, North Carolina

CHAPTER 1

The EMT and the Advanced Life Support Team

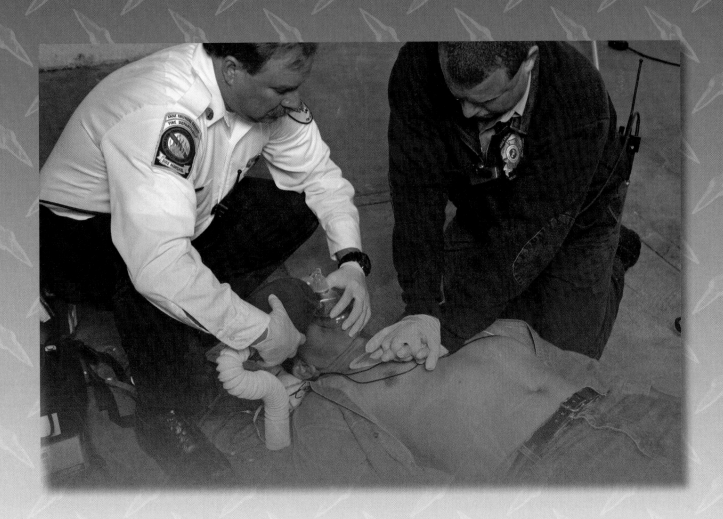

The purpose of this book, *ACLS for EMTs,* is to make you, as a practicing EMT, an even more valuable member of the emergency medical services (EMS) team. This material builds on the foundation of your initial EMT training and education by introducing or expanding your existing knowledge of pharmacology, ECG interpretation, electrical interventions, and airway management. You will learn how to contribute further to patient care efforts in each of the critical areas mentioned previously. Although completion of this course will not certify you to perform **advanced cardiac life support (ACLS)** skills in the field, the knowledge and understanding that you gain from this program will enhance the care you provide as well as the value that you bring to your EMS team.

Teamwork is the cornerstone of ACLS. Advanced life support (ALS) can only function on a foundation of solid, ongoing basic life support (BLS) practices. As such, an understanding of the principles of ALS will enhance your ability to work in collaboration to increase the survival rates of the patients that you serve. Most importantly, better teamwork will improve care not only during cardiac arrests, but also during all emergency calls.

■ Sudden Cardiac Arrest

During the next year, approximately 300,000 people in the United States will collapse from **sudden cardiac arrest**. Their hearts will stop beating, and without emergency cardiac intervention, they will die. Many of these victims will be assessed and treated by emergency medical personnel. Even with swift action, some will be too sick to survive; however, in some areas of the country, many of these victims (as many as 50%) will be resuscitated. These resuscitated victims of cardiac arrest will often go on to be discharged from the hospital neurologically intact and will be able to continue their lives thanks to the integrated continuum of dedicated care providers, from first responders to hospital staff.

But a continuum of care is more than just a collection of providers and equipment. Simply having resources available is not enough. **Emergency cardiac care** works best when applied with a systems

approach. Emergency cardiac systems of care bring together first responders, BLS and ALS EMS responders, emergency department physicians, nurses, cardiologists, and a host of allied health professionals in a coordinated team effort to improve outcomes for patients experiencing potential cardiac events. In fact, the integrated team approach is so important that it is a separate component of each and every ACLS program. But how does this work in the prehospital environment? Consider the following situations:

- The paramedic is unable to intubate a victim of cardiac arrest.
  - BLS ventilation continues to oxygenate the patient.
- A victim of cardiac arrest is defibrillated but the rhythm does not produce a pulse.
  - Quality CPR pumps blood and perfuses the heart and brain while resuscitation efforts continue.
- A patient calls 9-1-1 complaining of crushing chest pain. The transporting ambulance is 15 minutes away.
  - A BLS responder arrives first, applies oxygen, administers aspirin, and assists with the patient's nitroglycerin.

■ ALS and the EMT

The complexities of coordinating emergency cardiac care in the field bring into sharp focus the need for you to take your clinical education and apply it to practical situations. Nowhere is this more apparent than during a cardiac arrest. Few EMS personnel ever forget their first "code." They will often recall the difficulties that they encountered in vivid detail, highlighting the need for emergency cardiac care that can be applied practically in the field.

Although it is an unfortunate fact that the national average for successful resuscitation (discharge from the hospital neurologically intact) is somewhere between 2.5% and 20%, this does not mean that emergency cardiac care is ineffective. Rates in the area of 50% in some areas of the United

States that have established tightly coordinated systems of care highlight the room for improvement and the difference that a truly effective ALS/BLS team can achieve.

More than 15 years ago, EMS pioneer Peter Safar proposed changing the term CPR to CPCR (cardiopulmonary cerebral resuscitation) as a reminder that the brain, along with the heart and lungs, is an integral component of the resuscitation process.

At this point in time, medical science is unable to predict which patients can be successfully resuscitated. For patients who survive a sudden cardiac arrest, the ultimate goal for recovery is to return the patient as closely as possible to his or her former level of functioning and lifestyle. Because the brain is highly sensitive to lack of perfusion, cardiac arrest causes permanent damage to the brain more quickly than to other parts of the body. As a result, when a cardiac arrest occurs, the clock is ticking on your ability to resuscitate this patient in time to prevent brain damage. It is for this reason that EMS providers cannot wait to "figure out" how to work together to coordinate emergency cardiac care on scene. The team approach must be well coordinated before the call to ensure that, when the time comes to act, all personnel involved will provide the right care, the right way, at the right time, to resuscitate.

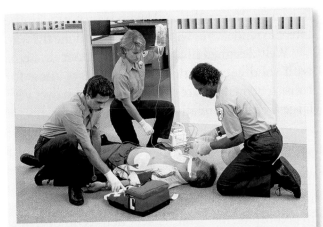

Figure 1-1 Members of the EMS team must work together to provide quality patient care.

■ BLS and ALS: The Team Approach

It is essential to understand that in the world of prehospital emergency care, BLS and ALS cannot exist without each other. BLS interventions may prevent sudden cardiac arrest, and if sudden cardiac arrest occurs, properly performed CPR and defibrillation are the core around which ACLS builds its resuscitative efforts. It would be a mistake to think of BLS care as only the "First Steps" of ALS care. Although BLS efforts begin early, they must continue throughout the continuum of care, carefully coordinated with the advanced tools and techniques being applied to stabilize and treat the patient's condition. Bringing BLS and ALS together in a seamless patient care endeavor requires focused effort, excellent communication skills, and solid teamwork. Each member of the EMS team must work in harmony with one goal in mind—quality patient care (**Figure 1-1**).

Many BLS systems implement what is referred to as a **tiered response model**, sometimes referred to as **ALS intercept** or **ALS rendezvous**. The goal of this type of system is to have a large number of BLS units (typically transport capable) while leaving a smaller number of ALS units (often nontransport units) available to respond only to calls for which ALS interventions are required. The benefits of a properly designed tiered response system are the following:

- BLS-equipped vehicles are cheaper to run than an all-ALS system.
- Larger numbers of BLS units typically allow for short response times between the 9-1-1 call and first patient contact.
- Although the ALS units typically have longer response times than the BLS units, they often arrive while the BLS crews are still performing their initial assessment and care.
- Reduced numbers of ALS providers allow for greater practice and experience in high-risk, low-frequency procedures and more direct medical oversight by EMS physicians.

Depending on the design of the tiered response system, the availability of ALS units, and the nature of the individual call, a BLS transport unit may elect to package the patient and begin transport with the intent to rendezvous with the ALS unit along the way.

Well-designed BLS/ALS tiered response systems with solid coordination between crews allow for consistent quality care to be delivered even over very large areas with relatively low call volume.

■ Goals for Patient Care

There are many ways for you and your team to improve patient survival. Everything that is done in prehospital medicine—every new technique, new intervention, protocol change, and standing order revision—should be motivated by a single question: Is this in the best interest of patient care? Only when the answer is "yes" will you truly be doing your best to meet the needs of our patients. With all this as the setting for your acquisition of additional knowledge and skills, the basics of emergency cardiac care will now be discussed.

When you are providing care to any cardiac patient, your energies should focus on the following (**Figure 1-2**):

- Reducing patient anxiety and decreasing pain
- Preventing **hypoxia**
- Maintaining adequate perfusion
- Coordinating with advanced levels of emergency cardiac care

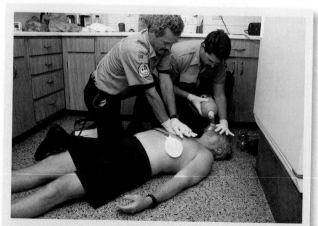

Figure 1-2   Quality patient care is the ultimate goal of every member of the EMS team.

It is vital for you to understand that these goals are interconnected. Failing in one is likely to undermine others, leading to poor patient outcome and possibly sudden cardiac arrest. For example, an anxious patient in severe pain has increased cardiac oxygen demands. If you know this and can lower the demands on the heart by reducing the patient's anxiety and pain, you can reduce the oxygen demand and avoid or reduce hypoxia, therefore preventing cardiac instability. If you do not recognize inadequate perfusion, there is an increased likelihood of cardiac damage.

■ Prevention of Sudden Cardiac Arrest in the Field

The best way to manage sudden cardiac arrest is to prevent it from occurring in the first place. Many patients encountered in the prehospital setting have the potential to deteriorate to the point of arrest; however, EMS providers will often arrive in time to intervene. In emergency cardiac care, this time frame is referred to as the **peri-arrest period**. It is critically important that effective BLS and ALS prehospital care be administered during the peri-arrest period because this is likely to influence the patient's ultimate outcome.

To prevent sudden cardiac arrest, your interventions need to be focused and implemented quickly. When a patient is scared or becomes stressed, the body reacts with a "fight or flight" response that unleashes a number of chemically active substances into the bloodstream. These substances cause the heart to beat faster and more forcefully. The increase in cardiac rate and strength of contractions means there is increased cardiac workload. As the workload of the heart increases, so does its need for oxygen to meet increased metabolic demands. If that oxygen need is not met, even briefly, the heart muscle progressively becomes more irritable and sudden cardiac arrest becomes more likely. When the patient is in this peri-arrest state, a problem that might be slight in another setting can cause sudden cardiac arrest in this setting.

Begin by making certain that the patient's airway is open and breathing and oxygenation are adequate. Once you have assessed the patient's level of consciousness and identified the chief complaint, try to ease the patient's anxiety. Being positive yet direct with your comments can help the patient relax. ("Mr. Matthews, we are going to take good care of you. Please try to relax and take some slow deep breaths of the oxygen.") Instill patient confidence by making clear that you are in control of the situation and have a plan of action.

Make the patient as comfortable as possible and discourage unnecessary movement. When the work of the body increases, so does the workload of the heart, thereby increasing the chance of cardiac damage or arrest. For example, if the patient says "I need to get my coat before I leave," respond by saying "Why don't you stay seated and tell me where it is and what it looks like, and I will get it for you?"

The patient's condition may require assessment or treatment that a BLS crew cannot provide. If you believe that the patient will require ALS interventions and ALS personnel are not already on scene, you will need to decide to either call them directly to the scene or package the patient and arrange for an ALS intercept or ALS rendezvous. It is tremendously important not to delay BLS care or transport to await the arrival of ALS personnel.

Before the ALS team arrives, auscultate the patient's breath sounds and obtain a complete set of baseline vital signs. Assess the patient using the OPQRST approach (onset, provoking factors/palliation, quality of pain, region and radiation of pain, severity, and time frames surrounding the event) presented in the chapter, *From Angina to AMI: The Cardiac Continuum of Care*. If possible and if time permits, obtain a SAMPLE history (signs and symptoms, allergies, medications, past history, last oral intake, and events leading up to the episode). Ask whether the patient has been prescribed medications and, if so, whether they have been taken as directed. Gather all the patient's medications and either take them to the hospital or turn them over to the responding ALS team. It is important to report baseline information to the incoming ALS team to better focus care provided by ALS and hospital personnel. By having all baseline information ready, you will speed up the patient handoff and the transfer of care to the ALS team.

Continually reassess the patient to determine whether his or her condition has changed and whether anything can be done to make the patient more comfortable. Keep the patient apprised as to what is going on. For example, you could say, "The paramedics will be here in just a few minutes. We just spoke with the physicians at the hospital and they are expecting you." Knowing that you have a plan and that it is coming together helps reassure your patient, which in turn helps reduce anxiety (**Figure 1-3**).

■ When the Patient Experiences Sudden Cardiac Arrest

If, despite your best efforts, your patient collapses while you are on the scene, it is easy to assume the cause to be sudden cardiac arrest. However, before you act on that assumption, be sure to assess the patient carefully.

The collapse may or may not be due to sudden cardiac arrest. A patient may lose consciousness for a variety of reasons. You need to perform all of the steps of a good BLS assessment to be sure you are giving your patient the most appropriate care.

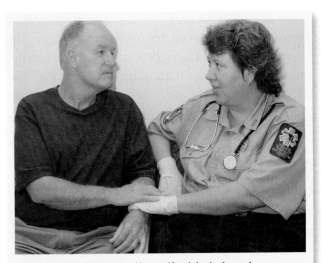

Figure 1-3   Reassure the patient to help reduce anxiety.

1. If the patient is unresponsive and not breathing or not breathing normally, call for additional help including ALS.
2. Get or call for an **automated external defibrillator (AED)** and apply it to the patient as soon as possible.
3. Begin chest compressions, pushing hard (2 inches on an adult) and pushing fast (a rate of at least 100 compressions per minute). Minimize interruptions in chest compressions for anything other than rhythm analysis or defibrillating with the AED.
4. Turn on the AED and apply the pads. AED administration is detailed in the chapter, *Electrical Interventions in Cardiac Care.*
5. When possible, move the patient to a long backboard or other patient transport device because this will simplify the move to the ambulance cot when it is time to transport the patient.

If an AED is readily available, it should be applied immediately and the rhythm analyzed. Studies have shown that up to 85% of victims of nontraumatic sudden cardiac arrest in the prehospital setting initially present in the shockable rhythms of either ventricular fibrillation (VF) or pulseless ventricular tachycardia (VT).

Rapid defibrillation can allow the heart to resume its normal electrical action quickly with a corresponding return of pulse and respirations. Your patient may even regain consciousness. The key to setting the stage for a successful defibrillation is performing outstanding, continuous CPR (ie, pushing fast and pushing hard with few, if any, interruptions).

■ What to Expect When ALS Arrives

Once on scene, the ALS team will reassess the patient. A significant part of that process will include obtaining a hand-off report from the BLS team. Be sure to provide a clear and concise report because it is imperative in good patient care. The information already gleaned from the patient assessment, the care that has been provided by the BLS team, and any additional information that is key to this specific patient should all be included in the hand-off report. A quality hand-off report is an important aspect of the patient care continuum and supports a team approach to patient care (**Figure 1-4**).

The hand-off report should be succinct. At a minimum, it should include the chief complaint(s), what has been done to address that complaint, and the extent to which your efforts have been successful. Identify all patient care interventions and the patient's response. Useful information includes such statements as "The patient was complaining of difficulty breathing but stated he had relief from oxygen" or "The patient reported that his chest pain was a 10 on a scale of 1 to 10, and it did not decrease despite administration of 15 L/min of oxygen for 6 minutes via a nonrebreathing mask." Keep in mind that valuable information does not necessarily equate with "good news." The ALS team must quickly ascertain which interventions have been performed and whether or not a difference was made in the patient's condition. Once the hand-off report has been completed and is given to an ALS provider, the ALS team assumes responsibility for patient care.

It is critical that the transition of care from BLS to ALS providers be as smooth as possible. For some BLS providers, making the change from running the call to being in a collaborative role can be difficult. A good way to facilitate the transition after completion of the hand-off report is to ask the ALS provider, "What else would you like us to do?"

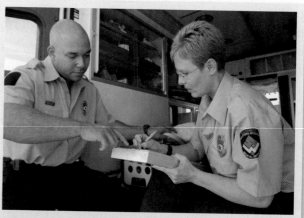

Figure 1-4 The hand-off report is an important aspect of the patient care continuum.

This makes it clear that you have handed off the patient and that he or she is now the responsibility of the ALS team.

While an ALS provider is taking the hand-off report, the other team member will often initiate ALS patient care measures at the same time. If the patient is not on a cardiac monitor, the paramedic will apply the cardiac monitor. If the need for a shock is confirmed, the paramedic will prepare to defibrillate the patient. As the EMT on hand, you may be needed to oxygenate the patient with a bag-mask device and 100% oxygen as the paramedic prepares to place an advanced airway. In some cases, you may be needed to prepare equipment while another ALS team member obtains IV access. ALS procedures like these are discussed in detail in the chapter, *Airway Evaluation and Control.*

If the patient is on a cardiac monitor when the ALS team arrives, electrodes may need to be changed or added so the paramedics can switch the patient over to their own monitor/defibrillator.

Another possible plan of action may be to initiate patient transport immediately and provide additional patient care en route to the hospital. In this case, you will need to prepare the cot, gather up any equipment, and make certain that the way to exit the emergency scene is clear.

In some EMS systems, if a patient has not been resuscitated after defibrillation, intubation, and several rounds of drug therapy, the decision to stop resuscitative efforts may be made. In that case, it may be necessary to contact the medical examiner or a funeral home. Check your local protocols for direction with regard to what EMS personnel should do in the event of patient death secondary to nonresuscitation. In this situation, make certain that family members or responsible parties are notified of the patient's death. Survivors on the scene will need gentle, caring support from the EMS team.

By working well together, the BLS and ALS team members can improve the quality of care being rendered as well as the efficiency with which the care is provided.

PREP KIT

■ Vital Vocabulary

advanced cardiac life support (ACLS) The provision of emergency cardiac care using invasive techniques or technology.

ALS rendezvous or ALS intercept A model for patient care in which the BLS team receives the call and arranges for ALS providers to meet them at an agreed-on location, resulting in providing ACLS care to the patient as soon as possible.

automated external defibrillator (AED) A small computerized defibrillator that analyzes electrical signals from the heart to determine when ventricular fibrillation is taking place and then administers a shock to defibrillate the heart.

emergency cardiac care The principles of emergency medicine focused specifically on a patient with a cardiac-oriented problem(s).

hypoxia A dangerous condition in which the body tissues and cells do not have enough oxygen.

peri-arrest period The period just before or after a full cardiac arrest when the patient's condition is very unstable and care must be taken to prevent progression or regression into a full cardiac arrest.

sudden cardiac arrest A state in which the heart fails to generate an effective and detectable blood flow; pulses are not palpable in cardiac arrest even if electrical activity continues in the heart.

tiered response model Dispatch of both ALS and BLS to the same call. This may involve an ALS rendezvous or a direct response to the emergency scene.

■ Cases

1. Your squad is dispatched to a man "feeling ill" at an extended care facility. On arrival, you find that your patient is in cardiac arrest. You initiate CPR and prepare to apply the AED when the charge nurse tells you she thinks the downtime on this patient was most likely between 5 and 8 minutes before 9-1-1 was called.

   Assuming that the nurse's time estimate is reliable, how would this extended downtime impact the likelihood of the patient being successfully resuscitated?

2. A response to a local restaurant for an "unknown medical" finds you caring for a 59-year-old man who reports crushing chest pain and difficulty breathing. The onset of symptoms was approximately 1 hour prior, and the patient received no relief from taking two of his nitroglycerin tablets. He has been treated for angina for the last 2 years but has never experienced such devastating chest pain.

   What are the main patient goals for all patients with cardiac emergencies?

3. You are transporting a 70-year-old woman to the emergency department for a complaint of abdominal pain. While you are obtaining a baseline blood pressure, the patient suddenly gasps and slumps forward in full cardiac arrest.

   As you initiate care for this patient, what are your main goals when managing cardiac arrest in the prehospital setting?

CHAPTER 2

Airway Evaluation and Control

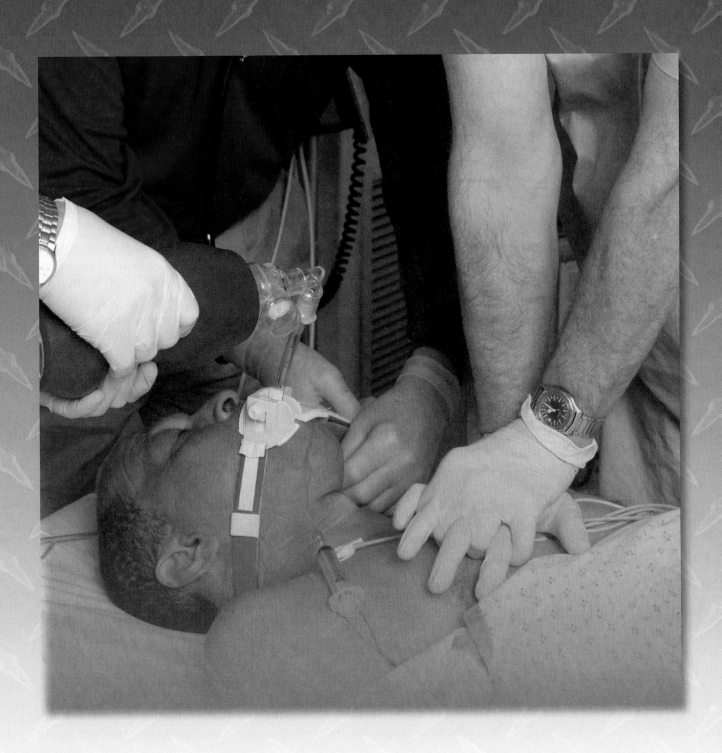

It is vital to understand that the goal of airway management is not simply to place an advanced airway; rather, it is a continuum of interventions ranging from use of a bag-mask device and an oropharyngeal airway (OPA) through the full spectrum of supraglottic airways (SGA) and adjuncts to direct placement of an endotracheal (ET) tube. Airway management is an ongoing process that requires continuous attention and may need to move in either direction along this continuum. For example, a bag-mask device may need to be replaced with a SGA. At other times, you may be able to avoid placement of an ET tube and continue management with a bag-mask device and an OPA airway.

Whereas the importance of maintaining a patent airway and ensuring adequacy of breathing cannot be overstated for any patient being cared for by EMS, you should remember that for patients in full cardiac arrest, airway management must never delay chest compressions. Cardiac arrest must be managed in a sequence of Compressions–Airway–Breathing (C–A–B). While this may seem to contradict the importance of airway management, what makes cardiac arrest a special situation can be explained by considering a patient's need for circulation as well as for respiration. If someone asked you to stand up right now, hold your breath, and walk across the room, could you do it? Yes, you could because although you have stopped breathing, your body continues to carry enough oxygen to let your metabolism continue for several minutes. Now, what if you were asked to stand, stop your heart, and then walk across the room? This is basically impossible because without circulation, the body's metabolism is interrupted almost immediately. This example shows why, when circulation is being provided by the body (the patient's heart is beating), airway management is virtually always the top priority. However, when circulation has stopped, you must reinitiate it manually with cardiopulmonary resuscitation (CPR) before airway management and ventilation (breathing) have any meaning.

You need to recognize the importance of airway and breathing management to ensure adequate ventilation and respiration in all your patients, not just those in cardiac arrest. Remember that respiration is a process that includes oxygen (O_2) transport and delivery as well as removal of carbon dioxide (CO_2) and other wastes. Of all the muscles in the body, the heart is one of the least tolerant of even brief interruptions in perfusion. To make matters worse, when a patient is in a cardiac-related crisis, the heart works harder and demands more oxygen. Typically, patients are anxious and frightened, and the actions of the **sympathetic nervous system** increase cardiac work and respiration demands.

This can occur no matter what is the precipitating event, whether it is angina or a myocardial infarction (heart attack). With any increase in cardiac workload comes a corresponding increase in cardiac oxygen needs. If the demand for oxygen is not met, tissue and blood oxygen levels (perfusion) decrease, and the heart becomes more ischemic, making it more irritable and electrically unstable. If oxygen inadequacy continues, this increased cardiac irritability will make the heart more likely to fibrillate, demonstrating on ineffective rhythm known as ventricular fibrillation (VF). Once in VF, the heart is no longer pumping effectively, and the patient goes into cardiac arrest.

It is for these reasons that patient airway and breathing adequacy is a top priority for EMS providers of all levels. Emergency airway management is the dynamic, almost circular, process of evaluating, managing, and reevaluating the patient to make certain that the airway remains patent and breathing is adequate.

The effective evaluation and control of your patient's airway and overall respiratory status can be broken down into three distinct yet related components:

- Anatomic
- Mechanical
- Chemical

Understanding how these three key components of respiration relate to each other will help you to control them effectively.

■ Anatomic Issues

The first step in maintaining an adequate airway is to ensure that air can move freely and without obstruction in and out of the patient. You must ensure that the airway is not closed off at any point by any part of the patient's airway anatomy or by a foreign object preventing movement of oxygen into and wastes out of the lungs.

Anatomic positioning is the foundation on which airway evaluation and control are built. As a general rule, patients who are conscious, alert, and spontaneously breathing are capable of protecting their own airways. Even a small piece of food falling on the epiglottis will stimulate a cough as the body instantly responds to keep the foreign body out of the airway and lungs. While foreign body airway obstructions do occur and must be addressed, the most common cause of airway obstruction is the tongue. In unconscious patients, the tongue muscles relax, the tongue falls into the back of the throat, and the patient can no longer protect the airway. Loss of muscle tone allows the tongue to fall backward into the pharynx, producing a variety of consequences ranging from sonorous respirations to complete obstruction of the airway (**Figure 2-1**).

In the absence of trauma, the most effective technique for opening the airway is the **head tilt–chin lift maneuver** (**Figure 2-2**). For an unconscious trauma patient with a suspected neck injury, the **jaw-thrust maneuver** is considered the best choice to spare the spine from further injury because it can be performed without unnecessarily bending the cervical spine by tilting the head back (**Skill Drill 2-1**). However, if either the head tilt–chin lift or jaw-thrust maneuver proves unsuccessful in producing an open airway, the head should be tilted back slowly until the airway is open and patent.

Positioning techniques should be used first when you are attempting to open an obstructed airway, because they can be used quickly and without any equipment. It would not be efficient to search for a piece of equipment when a minute or two could make the difference in whether or not the patient goes into respiratory or possibly even cardiac arrest.

For spontaneously breathing patients, simply correcting the position of the head, neck, and mandible may be all that is required to realign the anatomy and reestablish a patent airway. However, once that is accomplished, an airway adjunct such as an oropharyngeal or nasopharyngeal airway is often necessary to maintain the airway.

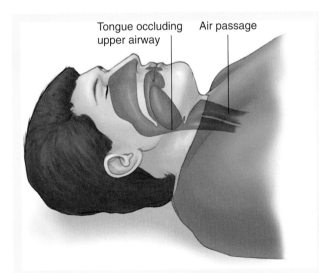

Figure 2-1 In an unconscious patient, loss of muscle tone allows the tongue to fall backward into the throat and block the airway.

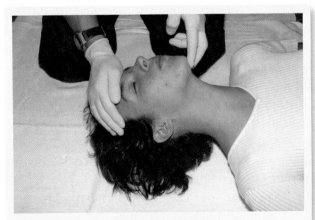

Figure 2-2 The head tilt–chin lift maneuver is a simple technique for opening the airway in a patient without a suspected cervical spine injury.

SKILL DRILL 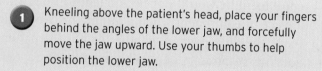 2-1   Performing a Jaw-Thrust Maneuver

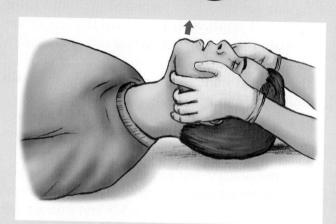

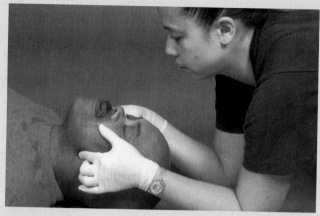

1 Kneeling above the patient's head, place your fingers behind the angles of the lower jaw, and forcefully move the jaw upward. Use your thumbs to help position the lower jaw.

2 The completed maneuver should look like this.

The use of suction also may be needed for maintaining airway patency. Complete airway obstruction can result when a patient's posterior pharynx is full of liquid or solid materials like blood, vomitus, or other matter. To make matters worse, materials like this in the airway may be aspirated, producing disastrous short- and long-term consequences. In the short-term, airway obstruction is of primary concern. In the long-term, patients who may be fortunate enough to survive but have aspirated blood or stomach contents into their lungs may develop aspiration pneumonia and/or adult respiratory distress syndrome (ARDS). Either condition greatly increases patient morbidity (incidence of disease) or mortality (incidence of death).

As an alert EMT caring for your cardiac patient, you should be quick to recognize the need for suctioning and have the equipment ready and available (**Figure 2-3**). Follow the steps in **Skill Drill 2-2**.

It is important to keep in mind common and serious complications of poor suctioning technique, including trauma, vagal stimulation (leading to dysrhythmias), and hypoxia.

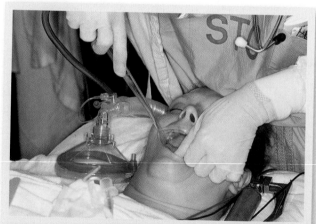

Figure 2-3   Suction any fluid or particles from the mouth before making any attempt to perform intubation.

SKILL DRILL　2-2　Suctioning a Patient's Airway

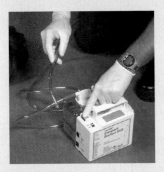

1 Make sure the suctioning unit is properly assembled and turned on.

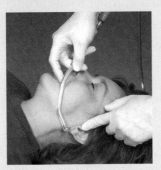

2 Measure the catheter from the corner of the mouth to the earlobe.

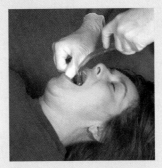

3 Open the patient's mouth and insert the catheter to the depth measured.

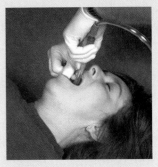

4 Apply suction in a circular motion as you withdraw the catheter. Do not suction an adult for more than 15 seconds at a time.

■ Mechanical Considerations

The process of breathing is a combination of two different mechanical events: inspiration and expiration. During inspiration, the normally dome-shaped diaphragm flattens and the muscles of the upper thorax expand, increasing the size of the chest cavity. When the chest expands in this way, it creates reduced intrathoracic pressure, causing air to be drawn into the lungs. During expiration, the muscles of the upper thorax relax, the chest wall returns to its normal position, and the diaphragm returns to its normal dome-like shape pushing out the air in the lungs. In this manner, inspiration is considered to be an *active process* when compared with the usually *passive process* of expiration, which normally takes about twice as long as inspiration.

It is important to note that the same reduction in intrathoracic pressure that draws air into the chest also helps blood return to the heart, thereby aiding in circulation. It is essential to understand that normal mechanical respiration works in this way as opposed to EMS provider-aided ventilation with a bag-mask device, which provides positive pressure to force air into the lungs, *increasing* intrathoracic pressure and *reducing* blood return to the heart. This point highlights the need to ensure that proper artificial ventilation may be beneficial for a patient, where excessive ventilation (rate or depth) may be harmful.

■ Chemical Processes/Gas Exchange

Open, patent airway anatomy and adequate mechanical ventalitory activity lead to the third component of respiration—the chemical process of gas exchange. With each inhaled breath comes another batch of oxygen-laden air, while each exhaled breath removes CO_2—the principal waste product of metabolism. This process must continue uninterrupted for the body to maintain an acid–base balance that is within the acceptable limits for biologic functions to continue. A patient's acid–base balance is measured as a blood pH, with a pH of 7.35 to 7.45 considered normal. A pH lower than 7.35 is considered acidosis, and a pH higher than

7.45 is considered alkalosis with pHs of 6.9 and 7.8 considered the extreme limits at which metabolism can continue and life can exist (**Figure 2-4**). When gas exchange does not occur in a portion of the lung, for example because of pulmonary edema or small airway collapse (atelectasis), a potentially lethal series of events begins. Instead of being able to cross the capillary membrane in the alveoli to then exit the body through exhalation, CO_2 remains in the blood, which then returns to the systemic circulation still loaded with CO_2 rather than with O_2. This retained CO_2 makes the blood more acidic. Therefore, as CO_2 levels rise, the pH falls (the body becomes increasingly acidotic), which interferes with metabolism, causing the heart to function less effectively. In addition, overall cellular function becomes less efficient.

When respirations are inadequate, the body has alternative means of meeting its metabolic needs. But because these means are less efficient, they produce greater quantities of more toxic metabolic waste, and acidosis worsens.

Understanding the anatomic, mechanical, and chemical requirements for adequate breathing is the first step in providing care for your patient. The next step is continually monitoring your patient to ensure that those requirements continue to be met the entire time that you have contact with your patient.

Evaluating the Adequacy of Breathing

Effective evaluation of breathing involves more than just counting breaths per minute and comparing that number to the normal baseline standard of 12 to 20 breaths per minute for adults (**Table 2-1**). In truth, your assessment needs to consider the rate of breathing as well as the depth of each breath and the work of breathing. A patient breathing at a rate of 10 breaths/min and taking slow, deep breaths may be exchanging O_2 and CO_2 efficiently. By comparison, a patient breathing at a rate of 18 breaths/min and taking shallow breaths may be in serious respiratory distress. Multiplying the respiratory rate times the depth of respirations (in mL) results in what is called minute volume. This is the amount of gas exchanged by the lungs each minute. For the average adult patient, minute volume usually is about 6,000 mL. Minute volumes of approximately 1,500 mL with a corresponding respiratory rate of

Table 2-1	Normal Respiration Rate Ranges
Adults	12 to 20 breaths/min
Children	20 to 30 breaths/min
Infants	25 to 60 breaths/min

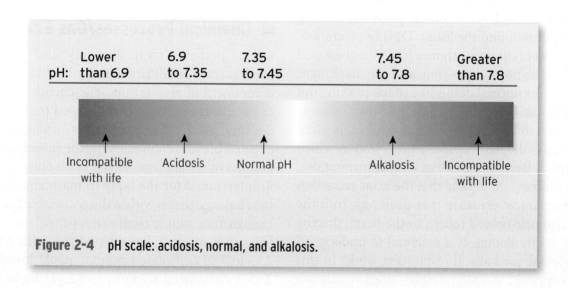

pH:	Lower than 6.9	6.9 to 7.35	7.35 to 7.45	7.45 to 7.8	Greater than 7.8
	Incompatible with life	Acidosis	Normal pH	Alkalosis	Incompatible with life

Figure 2-4 pH scale: acidosis, normal, and alkalosis.

between two and four breaths/min will only sustain life for several minutes.

The following steps should be taken to evaluate the adequacy of breathing:

- **Look at your patient's skin color**—A blue or gray tint usually indicates oxygen desaturation. Keep in mind that darker-skinned people often will first show signs of cyanosis in areas such as the nail beds, around the lips, earlobes, and/or the inner mucosa of the lips.
- **Assess the work of breathing**—Breathing usually is an automatic process that requires no thought or exertion. If a patient appears to be working hard at breathing, assume that there is a problem. Take immediate steps to identify and address the problem. Observe for accessory muscle use, retractions, and inability to speak in full sentences (ie, one- or two-word dyspnea), because each is a sign of increased work of breathing.
- **Listen to your patient's breathing**—The age-old maxim "Loud breathing is bad breathing" remains true today. Wet, gurgling sounds in the upper airway represent a potential life threat because of interference with air inflow. Wheezing or whistling breath sounds indicate reduced airflow through the smaller airways in the lungs, which in turn, results in a reduction in the amount of O_2 reaching the **alveoli**.

Patients may present with difficulty in breathing for many reasons during the peri-arrest period. Whereas many of these reasons may not be a result of cardiac problems, if left uncorrected, the hypoxia that results can lead to heart problems up to and including cardiac arrest. It is for this reason that, as an EMT, you will need to work with your BLS and ALS partners to ensure that your patient's airway and breathing are adequate while under your care.

■ Primary Adjuncts for Airway Control

Just as prehospital medicine has evolved, so has the potpourri of mechanical devices known as airway adjuncts. Even relatively simple devices like the ET tube are now available in many variations with a variety of features. There are many choices to be made as you attempt to improve the ventilation and oxygenation of your patient. Whereas oral and nasal airways may be considered "BLS adjuncts" and **endotracheal (ET) intubation** may be considered a "gold standard" of airway management, it is important to understand that your choice of airway adjunct will depend far less on your certification level than it will on the needs of the particular patient and circumstances that you are dealing with.

Bag-Mask Device

The bag-mask device has long been the device of choice for simple and effective ventilation by in-hospital and prehospital providers of all levels. There are a number of impediments to using a bag-mask device effectively, including beards and mustaches, facial fractures, displaced or misplaced dentures, obesity, and upper airway obstructions. However, the most common impediment is poor technique on the part of the bag-mask device operator—usually involving a poor mask seal or poor anatomic positioning.

Follow these steps for the two-person bag-mask device technique:

1. Kneel above the patient's head. If possible, your partner should be at the side of the head to squeeze the bag while you hold a seal between the mask and the patient's face with two hands. Pull the face up to the mask instead of pushing the mask onto the face.
2. Maintain the patient's neck in a hyperextended position unless you suspect a cervical spine injury, in which case you should immobilize the patient's head and neck in a neutral position and use the jaw-thrust maneuver. Have your partner squeeze the bag.
3. Open the patient's mouth, suction as needed, and insert an oral or nasal airway to maintain airway patency.
4. Select the proper mask size.
5. Place the mask over the patient's face, making sure that the top is over the bridge of the nose

and the bottom is in the groove between the lower lip and the chin. If the mask has a large round cuff around the ventilation port, center the port over the patient's mouth. Inflate the collar to obtain a better fit and seal it to the face if necessary.

6. Bring the lower jaw up to the mask with your last three fingers. This will help to maintain an open airway. Make sure you do not grab the fleshy part of the neck because you may compress structures and create an airway obstruction. If you think your patient may have a spinal injury, make sure your partner immobilizes the cervical spine as you move the lower jaw.

7. Connect the bag to the mask if you have not done so already.

8. Hold the mask in place while your partner squeezes the bag with two hands until the patient's chest visibly rises (**Figure 2-5**). If a spinal injury is suspected, immobilize the patient's head and neck with your forearms while maintaining an adequate mask-to-face seal with your hands. Continue squeezing the bag once every 5 to 6 seconds for adults and every 3 to 5 seconds for infants and children.

9. If you are alone, hold your index finger over the lower part of the mask and your thumb over the upper part of the mask, and then use your remaining fingers to pull the lower jaw into the mask. This is known as the EC-clamp method, and it will maintain an effective face-to-mask seal (**Figure 2-6**). Use the head tilt–chin lift maneuver to make sure the neck is extended. Squeeze the bag with your other hand in a rhythmic manner once every 5 to 6 seconds for adults and once every 3 to 5 seconds for infants and children.

10. Observe for gastric distention, changes in compliance of the bag with ventilations, and improvement or deterioration of the patient's condition.

TRAINING TIP

If you have a hospital or training program locally that has a respiratory therapy program, schedule an in-service session to receive advanced instruction in the use of bag-mask devices. While appearing to be simple devices, they are hard to use effectively, especially given the infrequency with which they are used in the prehospital setting.

Oropharyngeal Airways

The OPA is a curved device, usually made of plastic, designed to hold the tongue off the posterior aspect of the pharynx (**Figure 2-7**). It is only used in unconscious patients because it may stimulate

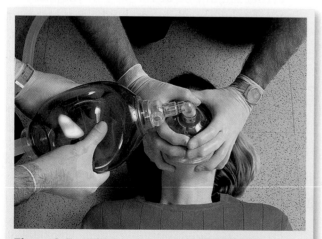

Figure 2-5   With two-person bag-mask device ventilation, you should hold the mask in place while your partner squeezes the bag with two hands until the patient's chest rises.

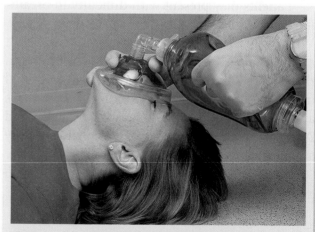

Figure 2-6   Maintain the seal of the mask to the face using the EC-clamp technique if you must ventilate alone.

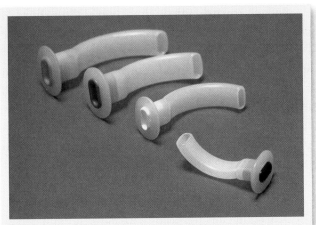

Figure 2-7 An oral airway is used for unconscious patients who have no gag reflex. It keeps the tongue from blocking the airway and makes suctioning the upper airway and posterior pharynx easier.

gagging, vomiting, and possibly even laryngospasm in the conscious or semiconscious patient.

OPAs are easily placed and, when in position, serve to facilitate suctioning as well. They also may be used to prevent intubated patients from chewing or biting on the ET tube.

Placing the correct size OPA is essential because one that is too large or too small will not function properly and may compromise the airway. The OPA is sized by measuring the distance from the corner of the patient's mouth to the angle of the mandible (earlobe) and comparing that to the distance from the flange to the distal tip of the OPA.

When trauma is not a factor, the OPA is placed by tilting the patient's head back and turning the device in a curve-up position (**Skill Drill 2-3**). After insertion has begun, and as the distal tip nears the posterior pharnyx, it should be rotated, allowing the curve of the device to follow the natural curve of the tongue.

Nasopharyngeal Airways

Unlike the OPA, which is only used in unconscious, unresponsive patients, the nasopharyngeal airway (NPA) can be placed in semiconscious patients (**Figure 2-8**). Ample lubrication prior to insertion reduces the likelihood of damaging the nasal mucosa and causing bleeding.

An NPA is a tubular device made of flexible rubber or plastic that usually is used when an OPA is too difficult to place or cannot be placed. Trismus (the inability to open the mouth fully), the presence of the gag reflex, or bleeding into the posterior

SKILL DRILL 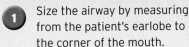 **2-3**   **Inserting an Oral Airway**

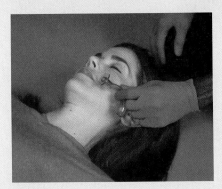

1 Size the airway by measuring from the patient's earlobe to the corner of the mouth.

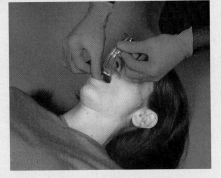

2 Open the patient's mouth with the cross-finger technique. Hold the airway upside down with your other hand. Insert the airway with the tip facing the roof of the mouth.

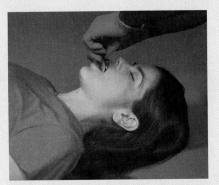

3 Rotate the airway 180°. Insert the airway until the flange (the trumpet-shaped flare) rests on the patient's lips and teeth. In this position, the airway will hold the tongue forward.

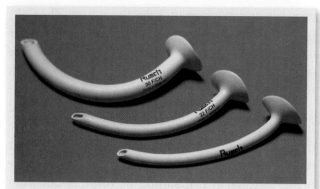

Figure 2-8 A nasal airway is better tolerated by patients who have an intact gag reflex.

pharynx that requires extensive suctioning are some examples of when an NPA might be a better choice of airway adjuncts.

Size the NPA by measuring from the tip of the nose to the patient's earlobe. As with the OPA, proper sizing is important. If the NPA is too long, it could extend partially into the esophagus. This should be suspected if you notice gastric distention or hypoventilation during ventilations, in which case the NPA should be removed and replaced with the next smaller size.

Lung sounds and the overall quality of ventilations should be reassessed after placing the NPA. Observe for gagging, vomiting, and laryngo-spasms when using an NPA on a responsive patient. Finally, be sure that the proper anatomic position is maintained whenever using an NPA by using the head tilt–chin lift method. In the case of a trauma patient, use of the jaw-thrust maneuver is preferred for maintaining the proper anatomic position.

Prior to insertion, the NPA should be well lubri-cated with a water-soluble lubricant. In some cases, the lubricant may include an anesthetic agent (usu-ally lidocaine). The NPA should be inserted gently, with even more care being required if it is made of plastic, because the rubber NPAs tend to be softer and more forgiving of the nasal mucosa (**Skill Drill 2-4**). The end of the nasopharyngeal airway is cut at a soft angle, and it can be rotated slightly if resistance is encountered during insertion.

Supraglottic Airways

Supraglottic airways (SGAs) come in a range of devices, each with their own features and varia-tions. Some of the most commonly used SGAs are

SKILL DRILL Inserting a Nasal Airway

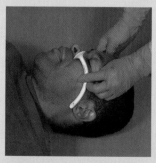

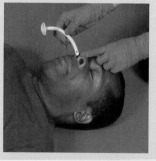

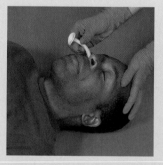

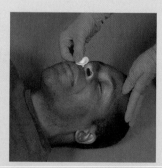

1. Size the airway by measuring from the tip of the nose to the patient's earlobe. Coat the tip with a water-soluble lubricant.

2. Insert the lubricated airway into the larger nostril with the curvature following the floor of the nose and the bevel toward the septum.

3. Gently advance the airway.

4. Continue until the flange rests against the nare. If you feel any resistance or obstruction, remove the airway and insert it into the other nostril.

the Easytube, the laryngeal mask airway (LMA), and the King LT airway (**Figures 2-9** and **2-10**). An advantage of SGAs is that they provide good protection and control of the patient's airway with rapid, simple, blind (does not require direct laryngeal visualization) insertion techniques that work well in a variety of difficult patient care circumstances.

When you are caring for a patient in cardiac arrest, insertion of an SGA can help improve airway control with minimal interruption of cardiac compressions. In fact, SGAs are considered equivalent to ET intubation for airway management during cardiac arrest (**Skill Drill 2-5**).

Weaknesses of SGAs include their sometimes incomplete seal on the airway that may not provide complete protection from aspiration and may not allow the generation of high pressures that may be required for the ventilation of some patients with poor lung compliance.

Endotracheal Intubation

In the world of airway control, the ET tube remains the gold standard. When a properly sized ET tube is placed and the cuff on the distal end is inflated, it isolates the airway completely, providing increased protection from aspiration of blood or gastric contents. In addition, the ET tube can also be used to deliver close to 100% oxygen, while allowing direct access for suctioning of the tracheobronchial tree.

ET tubes are available in various sizes and styles. Some tubes are equipped with inflatable cuffs to help seal the tube inside the trachea. Others do not have cuffs and rely on the provider placing the tube to closely approximate the diameter of the trachea and match it to the most appropriate-sized ET tube.

Placing an ET tube can range in difficulty from moderate to impossible, depending on certain variables, including anatomic features of the patient, the physical condition of the patient, and the circumstances under which the ET tube must be placed. Good hand-eye coordination, proper preparation, and good technique are the keys to a successful intubation.

In addition to the basic equipment carried by most ALS units, you may encounter specialized airway management equipment designed to make intubation faster, safer, and easier, especially under difficult circumstances.

Gum Elastic Bougie

The gum elastic bougie is a plastic stick, similar in appearance to the traditional ET stylet, only longer, more flexible, and with a slight bend at the very tip (**Figure 2-11**). This device is placed in a similar manner to the ET tube, except that being smaller and easier to maneuver, it can be much easier to insert in the trachea. In addition, bougie placement can

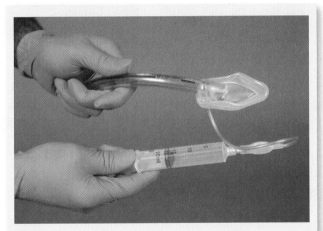

Figure 2-9   A laryngeal mask airway (LMA).

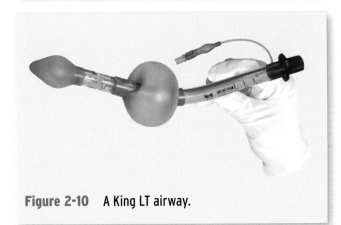

Figure 2-10   A King LT airway.

be confirmed by feeling the tip "rattle" across the cartilaginous rings of the trachea like a stick on a washboard, and by the fact that a bougie in the trachea cannot be inserted past the carina (the point at which the trachea splits into the right and left mainstem bronchi). Once the bougie is in place, an ET tube can be slid over it, perfectly following the bougie into proper position in the trachea.

SKILL DRILL LMA Insertion

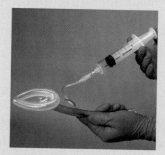

1 Take standard precautions. Check the cuff of the LMA by inflating it with 50% more air than is required for the size of airway to be used. Then deflate the cuff completely.

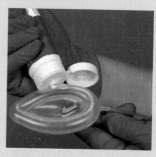

2 Lubricate the base of the device.

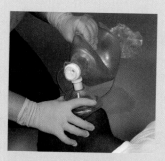

3 Preoxygenate the patient before insertion. Ventilation should not be interrupted for more than 30 seconds to accomplish airway placement. Place the patient in the sniffing position.

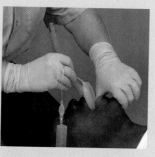

4 Insert your finger between the cuff and the tube. Place the index finger of your dominant hand in the notch between the tube and the cuff. Open the patient's mouth.

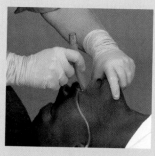

5 Insert the LMA along the roof of the mouth. Use your finger to push the airway against the hard palate.

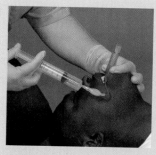

6 Inflate the cuff with the amount of air indicated for the airway being used.

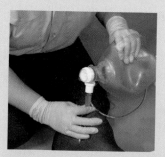

7 Begin to ventilate the patient. Confirm chest rise and the presence of breath sounds. Continuously and carefully monitor the patient.

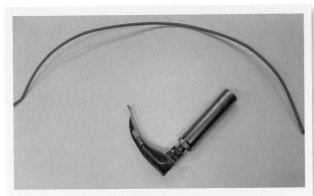

Figure 2-11 A gum elastic bougie shown next to a laryngoscope.

Lighted Stylet

A lighted stylet works much like a standard ET stylet, except that it has an extremely bright light at the very tip. Because the trachea is anterior to the esophagus, when the ET tube (and the lighted stylet) are in proper position, the bright light can be seen glowing in the throat from the outside of the patient, confirming the intubation. If the ET tube and stylet are improperly placed, the light will not be visible.

Video Laryngoscope

A variety of video laryngoscopes are available on the market ranging widely in price, features, and capabilities. The general feature that all such devices share is a tiny camera at the end of the laryngoscope blade, allowing an "inside" view of the trachea, vocal cords, and other structures of the airway to be seen on a screen attached somewhere on an outside portion of the device, usually the handle. In addition to facilitating intubation, these devices make excellent training aides both in the classroom as well as in the field.

Special Purpose Lighted Laryngoscope

Some laryngoscopes are available with special purpose and multilight systems that allow for improved visualization of airway structures.

Whereas a variety of ET facilitation devices are available, the basic technology involved with intubation is not complex. The laryngoscope is little more than a handle to which the laryngoscope blade is attached. The handle also serves as the place where the batteries used to illuminate the light source are kept.

Laryngoscope blades come in a variety of sizes and shapes that quickly snap on to the handle at a 90° angle. Each blade has either a tiny removable bulb or fiber optics at the distal end that serves to illuminate the key anatomic landmarks guiding the intubation.

The two basic choices of blades are straight (Miller) (**Figure 2-12**) or curved (Macintosh) (**Figure 2-13**). Other variations of blade types and styles can be found, but these are the two main types.

All providers should understand the intubation process because many of the steps required must be performed concurrently and in close coordination with each other. Whereas there are many individual steps involved in the preparation and practice of intubation, the process itself must occur quite rapidly. This highlights the need for cooperation between EMS providers of all levels to collaborate and not compete during advanced airway management or any other critical patient care skill. Some steps may differ depending on the specific equipment being used or the circumstances of the emergency call, but the core steps are outlined here.

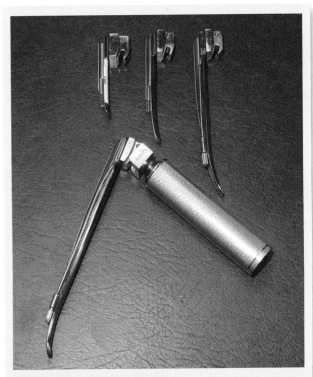

Figure 2-12 Miller blades.

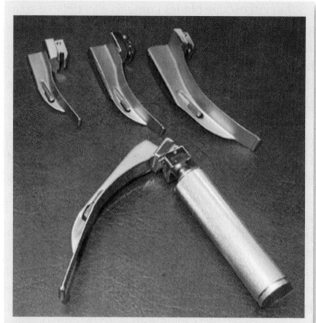

Figure 2-13 Macintosh blades.

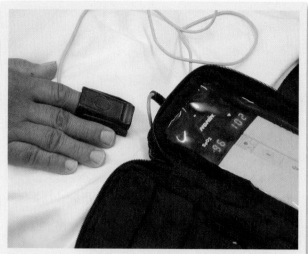

Figure 2-14 If a pulse oximeter is available, apply it so that the intubation can proceed once the oxygen saturation level is at 100%.

■ Preparing the Patient

BLS airway management should be established for the apneic patient and continued during set-up of the intubation equipment (**Figure 2-14**). This pre-oxygenation helps to ensure that the body has a residual supply of oxygen to draw on during the 10 to 30 seconds often required to place the ET tube, during which time no ventilations occur and the patient "desaturates." This desaturation can occur even more rapidly with particularly large and/or very sick patients, further reducing the time available for an intubation attempt.

Whereas many BLS airway management procedures will address difficult airway problems and facilitate intubation, it is important to keep in mind that if the patient has dentures, they should be left in place to assist with a bag-mask device seal, but removed for the intubation attempt to allow for a greater field of view.

All adult patients should be positioned with the head elevated to enhance alignment of the anatomic axes, ie, the sniffing position (**Figure 2-15**). In some cases, placing a folded towel under the head can further assist with positioning (**Figure 2-16**). Be prepared to assist with additional positioning or other

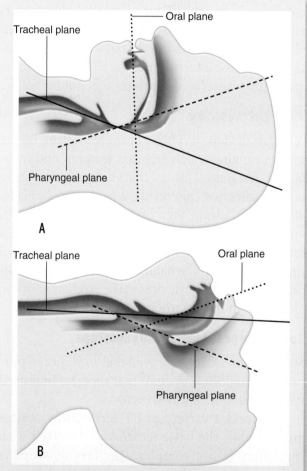

Figure 2-15 Three axes of the airway: oral, pharyngeal, and tracheal. **A.** Neutral position. **B.** Sniffing position.

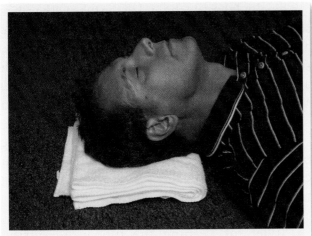

Figure 2-16   Head elevation is best achieved with folded towels positioned under the head.

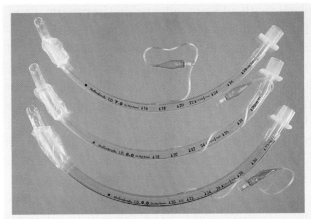

Figure 2-17   Endotracheal tubes that are most commonly used on adults generally range in size from 7.0 to 9.0 mm. Note the centimeter markings.

patient handling that may be necessary to manage specific difficult airway situations.

■ Preparing the Equipment

The correct style and size of laryngoscope blade should be selected based on the patient's age, anatomy, and size. The flange on the Macintosh blade helps control the tongue more easily than does a Miller. Most seasoned ALS providers have developed a preference for one style or another.

The notched area on the proximal end of the blade slides over the round bar on the top of the laryngoscope handle. Snap the two together to engage. As the blade is lifted up, it pivots on the bar and locks into place at a 90° angle. The light should illuminate when properly assembled. For blades with a removable bulb, the bulb should be checked to be sure it is "tight, white, and bright," or securely screwed in place and giving off a bright white light, which is your indication that there is ample power in the batteries. A dimly lit bulb indicates one of two things: either a potentially failing power source, in which case a different handle should be chosen or the batteries changed to prevent the light from failing during intubation, or the bulb itself is failing, in which case the bulb needs to be changed or a different blade used.

Next, select the correct size ET tube. As with all airways, ET tubes come in a variety of sizes based on the internal diameter of the tube (measured in millimeters) (**Figure 2-17**). Often, the person performing the intubation will request the size believed to be most appropriate based on the size of the patient's nostril or little finger. In addition to preparing the correct size, prepare one size smaller and one larger than requested. Also, take note of the horizontal marks placed at intervals down the length of the tube. These serve as reference points to gauge the depth of tube placement. When the tube is pushed to the corner of the mouth, the mark on the tube closest to that anatomic point should be identified. For an adult man, expect the tube to be at 21 to 23 cm, or 19 to 21 cm for an adult woman. These are only guidelines. Variations in neck length and jaw structure can alter anticipated depth levels, though they should not be markedly different. Once tube placement has been confirmed, you should periodically check your reference mark to help to ensure that the tube has not been pushed farther down into the trachea or possibly pulled out. In either case, the change in positioning must be noted and corrected.

Average ET tubes usually are 7.0 to 8.0 mm for an adult woman and 8.0 to 9.0 mm for an adult man. All adult size ET tubes are made of semi-rigid plastic with a 15-mm adapter on the proximal end. The adapter fits a variety of devices used to provide positive-pressure ventilation (**Figure 2-18**). ET tubes used on adult patients have a high-volume, low-pressure cuff near the distal end of the tube that is inflated after the tube is positioned. This is designed to seal the space that remains around the tube and to prevent air leaks during ventilations. It also reduces the risk of blood, vomit, or secretions making their way down the airway and being aspirated into the lungs. Attach a 10-mL syringe to the one-way valve, and insert about 8 to 10 mL of air to confirm that the cuff works and is not leaking. Assuming all is well, withdraw the air, at which time the cuff should deflate completely and collapse around the ET tube.

Whenever the cuff on an ET tube is inflated, the pilot bulb or balloon next to the one-way valve also will inflate. As long as the cuff remains inflated, the pilot bulb should remain firm. If the pilot bulb deflates, this signals that the cuff has failed and that the airway is no longer protected from aspiration. Should you notice this, immediately let the paramedic or ALS provider in charge of patient care know what has happened so he or she can take action.

Finally, lubricate the end of the tube with water-soluble jelly to facilitate a smooth pass of the tube and to help minimize damage to sensitive tissues, such as the vocal cords. Be sure not to use too much and occlude the openings on the end of the tube. When finished, you can use the tube packaging to ensure that the tube stays clean and ready for use.

After the laryngoscope handle and blade have been selected and checked, and the ET cuff has been checked and lubricated, assemble the following remaining equipment:

- Stylet for keeping the tube rigid during placement
- Water-soluble lubricant
- Suction unit with a large-bore tonsil tip in place
- Magill forceps for foreign body removal/aid to tube placement
- Esophageal detector devices
- End-tidal CO_2 detector (colorimetric device)
- End-tidal CO_2 waveform monitor (stand-alone unit or ECG monitor integrated)
- Stethoscope
- Bite block or oropharyngeal airway
- Tape or commercial device to secure the tube

Figure 2-18 The components of the adult ET tube include a 15-mm adapter that attaches to a ventilating device, a pilot balloon, the ET tube itself, an inflatable cuff (shown inflated), and the Murphy eye. The pediatric tube shown at the bottom includes an adapter and a Murphy eye at the uncuffed distal end of the tube.

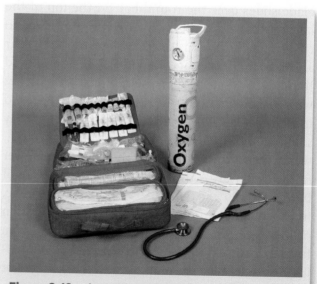

Figure 2-19 A complete airway kit.

- Cervical collar to restrict head/neck movement that may dislodge the tube
- Additional equipment as needed to facilitate difficult intubations:
  - Gum elastic bougie
  - Lighted stylet
  - Video laryngoscope
  - Special purpose lighted laryngoscope
  - Supraglottic airway

Figure 2-19 shows a complete airway kit.

■ Intubating the Patient

Once the patient is preoxygenated and all the equipment is ready, it is time to begin the intubation. In most cases, the EMT continues ventilating with the bag-mask device until the provider performing the intubation signals to stop ventilations.

As soon as ventilations cease, the laryngoscope is held in the left hand and gently inserted into the mouth from the right side, sweeping the tongue to the left, and moved into position in order to visualize the landmarks of the airway (**Figure 2-20**).

The tongue is swept to the left, and as the blade reaches midline, it is advanced toward the posterior pharynx. Be prepared to suction or to hand the intubator the suction catheter if the situation warrants. If a straight blade is being used, the epiglottis is lifted

directly. By comparison, if a curved blade is being used, the distal tip is inserted into the vallecula (the area between the base of the tongue and the epiglottis), and the epiglottis is lifted indirectly (**Figure 2-21**). The EMT may be asked to manipulate the cricoid cartilage [external laryngeal manipulation (ELM), also known as bimanual laryngoscopy] (**Figure 2-22**). This is accomplished by placing two fingers over the cricoid membrane (Adam's apple) and gently pushing down toward the patient's back as well as slightly to the patient's right up toward

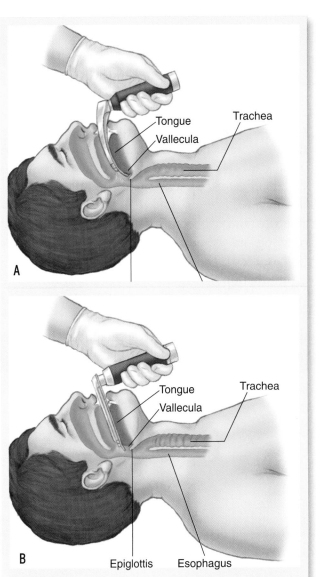

Figure 2-21 **A.** Insert a curved blade just in front of the epiglottis into the vallecula. **B.** Insert a straight blade past the epiglottis.

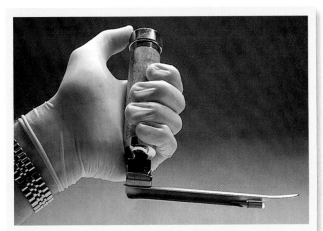

Figure 2-20 The laryngoscope is held in the left hand, and the blade is inserted in the right side of the mouth.

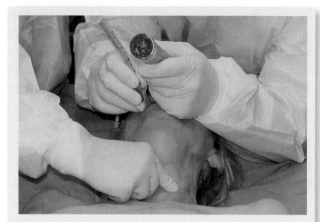

Figure 2-22   External laryngeal manipulation or bimanual laryngoscopy.

the patient's head, as directed by the intubator. This technique improves the visualization process by bringing the trachea and the surrounding structures into view. In addition, the EMT performing ELM may feel the tube actually pass through the vocal cords, which are directly below the EMT's fingers. If this occurs, he or she should let the intubator know.

After the epiglottis has been lifted, the glottic opening and the vocal cords should come into view (**Figure 2-23**). These are the key landmarks during an intubation. Without clear visualization of the vocal cords, the insertion of an ET tube is termed a "blind intubation" that will most likely result in the tube passing into the esophagus rather than the trachea.

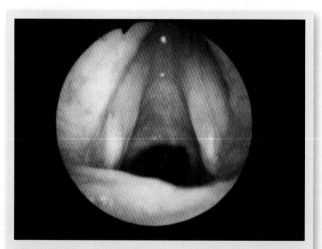

Figure 2-23   A view of the vocal cords.

After visualizing the key landmarks, the tube is inserted *and should be seen passing through the vocal cords*. The laryngoscope is gently removed from the patient's mouth, avoiding any contact with the teeth or lips. If a stylet was used, it is removed at this time. At this point, look for the mark on the ET tube in reference to the edge of the patient's teeth or gums. The cuff will be inflated and the syringe removed, during which time the EMT should reattach the bag-mask device and begin to ventilate the patient. Expect to provide at least three ventilations, so that equal breath sounds over each lung can be confirmed as well as the absence of sounds over the epigastrium. Do not overinflate the lungs, and allow adequate time for exhalation. Recheck breath sounds after cuff inflation. Nothing should be heard over the stomach. Bubbling or gurgling over the stomach, absence of chest wall movement, and absence of breath sounds all point to an esophageal intubation.

At least two other methods should be used to confirm correct placement of the ET tube. These may include the following:

- Observing for fogging of the tube
- Esophageal detector device
- Increase in pulse oximeter reading
- Positive CO_2 colorimetric device reading (yellow)
- End-tidal CO_2 waveform monitoring

Whereas direct visualization of the ET tube passing through the vocal cords is the best method of confirmation, end-tidal CO_2 waveform monitoring is the best noninvasive method of ensuring that the ET tube is in the correct position. Readings should produce a good waveform with each ventilation and should be at least 10 mm Hg during CPR and between 35 and 45 mm Hg for a patient with a pulse. In addition, this is an excellent method of monitoring the quality of CPR.

It is critically important to recognize esophageal intubation. If the esophagus has been inadvertently intubated, reattach the syringe, deflate the cuff, and remove the tube. Ventilate the patient for at least 30 seconds in order to preoxygenate the patient before another intubation attempt. In addition, time should be taken by the entire EMS crew to work together to address the issues that are making the intubation difficult. Simply reattempting intubation or switching intubators is not an effective method to deal with a failed intubation attempt.

Once correct placement has been confirmed, secure the ET tube by using a commercially available device. In some systems, an OPA is placed beside the ET tube to serve as a bite block should the patient begin to breathe on his or her own. Breath sounds should be checked again, as well as the reference mark on the side of the tube next to the corner of the patient's mouth. As the EMT continues to ventilate the patient, the mark should be checked periodically to make certain the tube does not move (pull out or slip down). If the ET tube has been pushed down, it will usually enter the right mainstem bronchus. This is most easily confirmed if breath sounds are present on the right side and absent or diminished on the left side or if oxygen saturation levels begin to fall on the pulse oximeter. Should this occur, it is best to deflate the cuff partially and gently pull the tube back about $1/2$ inch, while simultaneously ventilating and rechecking breath sounds. If bilateral breath sounds reappear, the cuff should be reinflated, the tube resecured, and ventilations resumed. Care should be taken to avoid withdrawing the tube too far and having it come out of the trachea because it requires restarting the whole intubation process, not

to mention leaving the airway unprotected. In many cases, a repeat intubation is harder than the first, so inadvertent extubation should be avoided.

The actual intubation—from cessation of ventilations to giving the first breath to confirming proper placement—should not take any more than 30 seconds; during cardiac arrest, 10 seconds is preferable.

As long as the respiratory or cardiac arrest continues, the intubated patient should be ventilated every 6 to 8 seconds without pauses in compressions. As previously discussed, *ventilating at rates faster than this will not benefit the patient* and will, in fact, decrease circulation by reducing blood return to the heart.

With proper technique and ideal circumstances, ET intubation can be performed without complication. However, complications do occur and can include lacerations of the lip or tongue, chipped teeth, soft-tissue damage, and tracheal swelling or bleeding. The most common reasons for failure to successfully intubate are inadequate assessment and preparation.

■ Cricothyrotomy

In some cases, the EMS team may be unable to place an ET tube or an SGA, or unable to ventilate with a bag-mask device. In these extreme cases, the only remaining option is to create an artificial opening in the throat called a cricothyrotomy. Cricothyrotomy is only used as a last resort in airway management.

PREP KIT

■ Vital Vocabulary

alveoli The grape-like clusters of air sacs of the lungs in which the exchange of oxygen and carbon dioxide takes place.

endotracheal (ET) intubation Insertion of an endotracheal tube directly through the larynx between the vocal cords and into the trachea to maintain and protect an airway.

head tilt–chin lift maneuver A combination of two movements used to open the airway by tilting the forehead back and lifting the chin; used for nontrauma patients.

jaw-thrust maneuver Technique to open the airway by placing the fingers behind the angle of the jaw and bringing the jaw forward, which in turn pulls the tongue forward as well; used when a patient may have a cervical spine injury.

sympathetic nervous system The part of the autonomic nervous system responsible for defensive, compensatory responses; often called the fight-or-flight system.

■ Cases

1. A man collapses at a high school football game and is found to be in full cardiac arrest. He is shocked three times without converting to an organized rhythm, and CPR continues as you await the arrival of ALS. Once on scene, the paramedic is preparing to intubate and asks you to preoxygenate the patient as he prepares his equipment.

What is the purpose of preoxygenation?

2. You respond to the local YMCA where you find an 80-year-old man unconscious and unresponsive in the dining hall. As you approach, you see that his head is slumped forward on his chest and that he is extremely cyanotic.

What does the patient's skin color imply? How should you initially manage this patient's airway problem?

3. EMS is called to a private residence and arrives to find a 62-year-old man in acute respiratory distress. The patient has a long cardiac history. His wife tells you that he may have accidentally taken too many painkillers given to him for a recent foot surgery. You notice that the patient appears to be breathing approximately 6 times a minute and the breaths are shallow.

How can this respiratory situation adversely impact this patient's cardiac condition? What is your initial focus relative to this patient's respiratory status?

CHAPTER 3

From Angina to AMI: The Cardiac Continuum of Care

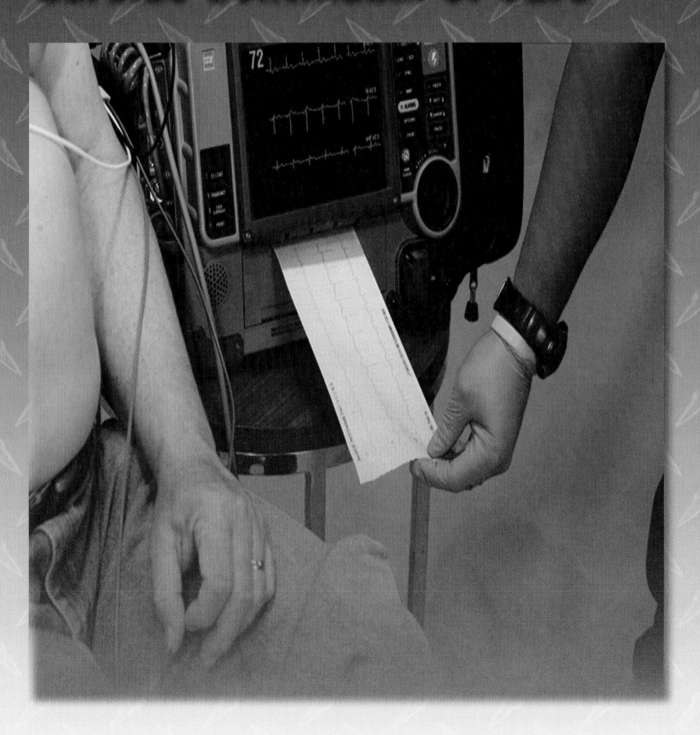

More than 1.25 million heart attacks occur in the United States every year at a cost of over 100 billion dollars. Heart disease causes almost one in every four deaths in North America. Of these, almost half occur outside of the hospital.

The severity of a medical problem such as this raises the question, "What can EMS do about it?" The answer lies in being able to understand and intervene in the **cardiac continuum of care**. The cardiac continuum of care is the collection of all of the different resources and services required to care for someone with heart disease.

EMS plays a key role in this cardiac continuum of care because providers are often the first point of contact when signs and symptoms of an acute cardiac condition become obvious.

In addition, this chapter discusses how EMS coordinates with other parts of the continuum in what is called **systems of care**, or how all of the parts actually work together. In some systems, the integration and coordination is flawless between the different parts of emergency medical services, from first responder to paramedic interaction and coordination with different parts of the hospital from the emergency department to the cardiac catheterization lab. This text strives to help all types of prehospital care providers work together to provide optimal assessment and treatment in the cardiac system of care to allow for the best possible outcome for the patient.

For many patients, the first symptom that will lead them to call 9-1-1 and enter the cardiac system of care will be chest pain (**Figure 3-1**).

■ The Progression of Cardiac Disease

The onset of the pain or discomfort of **angina** is usually associated with exertion or stress of some kind and may be described as a dull, squeezing feeling, tightness, or pressure in the chest. Patients who are experiencing classic angina are commonly diaphoretic and may have additional complaints of difficulty breathing or shortness of breath, and possibly be nauseated or vomit. Patients may allude to having heart palpitations, sometimes saying that they feel like there are "butterflies in their chest" or that their "heart is racing." In the absence of a medical background, keep in mind that patients will draw from their vocabulary and life experience to describe what they perceive is happening. You may hear comments such as "I just feel different" or "I have this funny feeling." Again, you must be able to interpret their words into medical terms. Avoid the danger of discounting the potential severity of a patient's condition simply because the patient does not use accurate medical terminology.

As coronary disease progresses over time, the angina a patient experiences may eventually become unstable. When this occurs, there is typically a change in the pattern. Patients may experience an increase in the frequency or length of their episodes or attacks as well as in the degree of pain or discomfort being experienced. Although exertion may still precipitate the problem, patients may not recognize

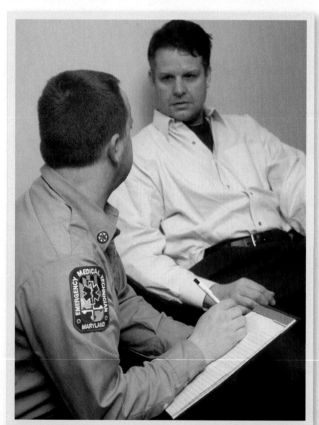

Figure 3-1   The chief complaint is the patient's initial response to the question "What's wrong?" or "Why did you call 9-1-1 today?"

Table 3-1	Signs and Symptoms and Other Indicators of Acute Coronary Syndromes			
Classic Symptoms	**Atypical Symptoms**	**Anginal Equivalent Symptoms**	**Risk Factors**	
Crushing chest pain	Stabbing pain	Shortness of breath	>65 years of age	
Pain in the center of the chest	Pain that changes on movement or palpation	Diaphoresis	Known CAD	
Pain radiating to the left arm	Epigastric pain	Near syncope	Diabetes	
			Hypertension	

the seemingly small activity preceding the attack as exertion. You may hear a patient say "I just went out to the porch to get the paper, and I couldn't catch my breath."

Complaints of fainting, weakness, dizziness, or confusion should be taken seriously in all patients because they may be precursors to a serious cardiac event. With the progressive worsening of the patient's condition that moves the person into the **unstable angina** category often comes an increase in the severity of the attacks or episodes. Failure of rest or prescribed medications (usually nitroglycerin) to relieve the patient's symptoms indicates a heart in need of oxygen and a delivery system that is incapable of meeting that basic metabolic need. With increasing cardiac ischemia and **acute myocardial infarction (AMI)**, sudden cardiac arrest may be imminent.

As such, you must be able to identify patients in need of entry into the cardiac continuum of care well before they get to the point of obvious AMI or cardiac arrest. Doing so requires you to recognize not only classic "anginal" chest pain, but also atypical pain (such as stabbing, pleuritic, or positional pain), anginal equivalents (diaphoresis, shortness of breath, syncope), and risk factors such as positive family history, known **coronary artery disease (CAD)**, hypertension, and diabetes mellitus (**Table 3-1**).

■ Assessment of the Cardiac Patient

Without question, identifying the chief complaint and obtaining an accurate history are key contributions that can be obtained by EMTs in the field setting. Of the common chief complaints (**Table 3-2**), chest pain or discomfort is most commonly associated with AMI, although it is important to keep in mind that many other complaints, when combined with further assessment, may lead to a patient's inclusion in the cardiac continuum of care and treatment for cardiac issues. One of the keys to obtaining an accurate history in as short a time as possible is to use a standardized approach. This ensures that all the right questions are asked. An initial SAMPLE history will enable you to obtain much pertinent information in a short period of time under a wide variety of circumstances (**Table 3-3**). Once the SAMPLE history is obtained, assessment questions focused on the patient's complaint may follow the OPQRST

Table 3-2	Common Chief Complaints

- Chest pain/pressure
- Indigestion
- Discomfort
- Difficulty breathing
- Weakness
- Fainting
- Palpitations
- Squeezing
- Tightness

Table 3-3	SAMPLE Medical History
S	Signs and symptoms of the injury or illness. These should be the reasons that caused the patient to call for emergency medical services. Patients should describe signs and symptoms in their own words.
A	Allergies. Patients may be allergic to medications, food, or airborne particles.
M	Medications. What medications is the patient taking? Ask about medications prescribed by the patient's physician, over-the-counter (nonprescription) medications, and herbal remedies.
P	Pertinent past medical history. What events or symptoms might be related to the patient's current illness? For example, it would be important to know whether a patient experiencing severe chest pain had a previous heart attack.
L	Last oral intake. When was the last time the patient had anything to eat or drink? Find out what the patient last ate or drank and how much he or she consumed.
E	Events associated with or leading to this injury or illness. Knowing these events will help you put together the pieces of the medical history puzzle. Let patients describe these events in their own words.

acronym, which is typically used when assessing a patient reporting pain or discomfort (**Table 3-4**).

Given the basic templates of SAMPLE and OPQRST, you can use the same basic questions to elicit a history based on a complaint of difficulty breathing, weakness, discomfort, or even feeling funny. In fact, with simple modifications, you can use these tools with virtually any chief complaint. This will allow you to quickly gather important information, which in turn, will help you identify and prioritize the most pressing problems, allowing you to facilitate a better care plan.

Table 3-4	The OPQRST of Pain

O—Onset
   Key Question: What were you doing when the pain/discomfort started?

P—Provoke/Palliation
   Key Question: What makes the pain/discomfort better or worse? What have you tried to reduce the symptoms? Nitroglycerin? Antacids? Rest? Did they work?
   Support Questions: Has this ever happened before? If so, when?

Q—Quality
   Key Question: What does the pain feel like (squeezing, burning, heaviness)?

R—Region/Radiation
   Key Question: Can you point with one finger to the main area of pain/discomfort?
   Support Questions: Do you feel pain anywhere else? If so, can you show me or tell me where it is?

S—Severity
   Key Question: How bad is the pain on a scale of 1 to 10, with 1 being no pain and 10 being extreme pain?
   Support Questions: What is the worst pain you've ever experienced? How does this compare?

T—Time Frames
   Key Question: When did you first notice the symptoms?
   Support Questions: Have the symptoms been continuous? If not, has the feeling come and gone?

Another good model to incorporate into your patient assessment is the four-phase assessment approach. This approach lets you consider the information that you will be collecting to use in your assessment in four distinct phases. This method can help you keep in mind that a sound assessment continues throughout each and every phase of the emergency call (**Table 3-5**).

You should start the process of assessing your patient from the moment you are dispatched to the call. The process continues as you approach the patient and then make direct contact and introduce yourself and your partner. When you shake the patient's hand and feel for a pulse, you also can assess the patient's skin condition. Then look in your patient's eyes and take note of any verbal response or gesture relative to your entry. This process of assessment will continue through your SAMPLE and OPQRST questions, your physical assessment of the patient, vital signs, and additional information that you may be able to gather directly from the scene itself. As a continuous process, your assessment will go on through your transport of the patient and will only end when you summarize your findings in a clear and concise hand-off report.

■ Key Concepts of Emergency Cardiac Care

As described in the chapter *The EMT and the Advanced Life Support Team*, there are four fundamental goals in emergency cardiac care. These goals reach across the borders of field medicine into the hospital setting. EMTs, AEMTs, paramedics, nurses, and physicians must work collectively to meet these goals and contribute to the success of the overall patient care effort.

1. **Reduce Pain and Anxiety**—Various analgesics and anxiolytics are used to reduce pain and anxiety in cardiac patients. Morphine, fentanyl, or self-administered nitrous oxide can all provide analgesia for a cardiac patient. Lorazepam and other anxiolytics can be administered to help alleviate anxiety. The reduction in a patient's pain and anxiety can lead directly to a reduction in myocardial

---

Table 3-5   The Four-Phase Assessment Approach

Phase 1—En Route

Includes early dispatch information and initial scene presentation on arrival, including the nature of the call (chest pain, shortness of breath, and syncope are all examples of incidents that may be cardiac in nature). The location to which you are dispatched can also provide context about the patient's condition (private home, physician's office, business, extended care facility). The initial scene presentation can clue you in about the patient's ongoing medical care and activities of daily living (ADLs), which are important aspects of patient history.

Phase 2—Approach

Includes the approach up to first patient contact and primary assessment. In addition to scene safety, this phase includes the early assessment of transport priority. That is, the sick/not sick decision for immediate transport, or further assessment on scene. This is also the point at which airway, breathing, and circulation are assessed for immediate life threats.

Phase 3—Patient

Includes direct patient contact including the rapid or focused assessments as necessary. This phase may include a rapid medical history (SAMPLE) and vital signs as well as focused questioning (OPQRST) about the patient's signs and symptoms and complaints.

Phase 4 –Transport

This phase may begin before actual patient transport can be achieved and includes ongoing assessment with more detailed questioning and physical exam as needed. This phase also includes assessment of the adequacy of interventions. That is, an assessment to decide if your interventions are helping or harming and if they need to be continued as is, modified, or discontinued.

oxygen demand and, possibly, improved outcomes. While ALS personnel may administer medications to help accomplish this goal, providers of every level have the responsibility to manage the emergency scene and communicate with the patient in such a way as to help the patient relax and reduce his or her oxygen demand.

With increased or ongoing dosing of narcotics like morphine or fentanyl comes an increased risk of central nervous system and respiratory depression. You must be alert for .any changes in the patient's level of consciousness and must continually evaluate the adequacy of breathing (**Figure 3-2**). Be prepared to quickly step in and assist with ventilations should the need arise.

Fentanyl is a synthetic narcotic more powerful than morphine. It does not depress respirations as much as morphine and, as such, is considered to be the analgesic of choice in many systems.

2. **Prevent or Correct Hypoxia**—You should initiate oxygen therapy if the patient is truly hypoxic ($Spo_2 < 94\%$) or if you suspect that the patient is being deprived of oxygen for any reason (**Figure 3-3**). Although a nasal cannula may be less restrictive and seemingly better tolerated by the patient, the concentrations of delivered oxygen using that particular device are relatively low—a maximum of about 36%. Whether the patient presents with the anxious, skittish behavior often found with early hypoxia or the markedly decreased level of consciousness associated with more serious levels of hypoxia, corrective intervention needs to occur as soon as possible. Pulse oximetry should be used to determine oxygen levels in the blood and oxygen administration tailored to the patient's need. To that end, 12 to 15 L/min of oxygen delivered via a nonrebreathing mask will deliver close to 100% oxygen and reverse the hypoxia quickly. For the patient who seems hesitant to use the mask, direct yet empathetic communications to encourage its use often will result in patient compliance. The mask allows you to deliver almost three times the concentration of oxygen as a nasal cannula and will raise the saturation levels quickly.

3. **Maintain Adequate Perfusion**—The use of various nitrate preparations has been repeatedly shown to be beneficial in emergency cardiac

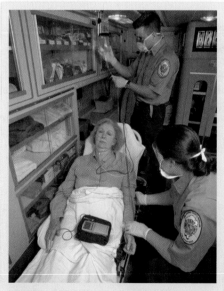

Figure 3-2 With increased or ongoing dosing of narcotics, you need to be alert for any changes in the patient's level of consciousness and must continually evaluate the adequacy of breathing because it commonly becomes slower and more shallow.

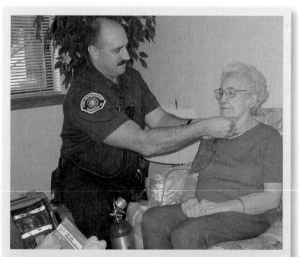

Figure 3-3 Oxygen therapy should be initiated by the EMT when oxygen levels indicate a need or if the patient is being deprived of oxygen for any reason.

care (**Figure 3-4**). Improved blood flow to the heart, specifically to the areas immediately surrounding the infarct or ischemic tissue, is the primary goal. Peripheral vasodilatory effects help to decrease the workload of the left ventricle, which directly reduces the heart's oxygen consumption. At the same time, nitrates increase coronary blood flow, which also is very desirable. In addition to nitrates, the prehospital administration of aspirin has been shown to improve outcomes for cardiac patients. Aspirin is recommended as soon as possible after onset of symptoms; it is suggested that dispatchers direct cardiac patients without contraindications to take it even before EMS arrives. With more and more EMTs having the capability to administer nitroglycerin and aspirin, delivery of these key cardiac medications should not be delayed. Irrespective of who administers nitrates, the patient's blood pressure needs to be carefully monitored to prevent it from becoming too low. In most protocols, the patients' systolic blood pressure needs to remain >100 mm Hg for nitrates to be safely administered.

You should obtain frequent blood pressure measurements when patients are receiving nitrates and more frequently if any drugs are being administered via the IV route.

4. **Coordinate with Advanced Cardiac Care**—Expect ALS or hospital staff to use drugs called beta-blockers for many patients with suspected AMI. This family of drugs has the ability to decrease heart rate, lower systolic blood pressure, and block the effects of the sympathetic nervous system, which makes them good choices in cardiac care. Again, you can positively contribute to patient care by being aware of a patient's vital signs and level of consciousness whenever these drugs are being administered (**Figure 3-5**). If changes in the patient's condition are noted, make certain that this information is passed on to the ALS team. For example, indicate that the patient is no longer responding when spoken to or that he or she has sonorous respirations.

As with most emergency medicine, excellent patient assessment skills and a focus on performing the basic components of patient care as flawlessly as possible will help to ensure the best outcome for the patient. Early access to ALS whenever possible and/or rapid, safe transport to the appropriate facility are essential considerations, as well. Finally, never forget that it often is the team's cohesiveness and ability to communicate effectively that may have the greatest effect on the success of its efforts.

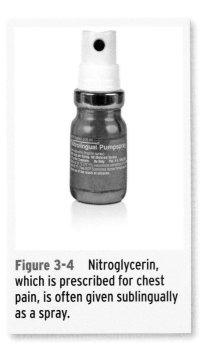

Figure 3-4 Nitroglycerin, which is prescribed for chest pain, is often given sublingually as a spray.

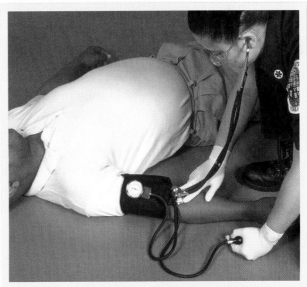

Figure 3-5 The EMT can positively contribute to patient care by continuously monitoring the patient's vital signs and his or her level of consciousness.

■ Vital Vocabulary

acute myocardial infarction (AMI) Heart attack; death of heart muscle following obstruction of blood flow to it. Acute in this context means "new" or "happening right now."

angina Transient (short-lived) chest discomfort caused by partial disruption of blood flow to the heart muscle.

cardiac continuum of care The collection of all of the different resources and services required to care for someone with heart disease.

coronary artery disease (CAD) Condition that results when atherosclerosis or arteriosclerosis is present in the arterial walls.

systems of care How EMS coordinates with other parts of the continuum of care and how all of the different parts actually work together—from EMS first responder to paramedic intercept to their coordination with the hospital and emergency department cardiac catheterization lab.

unstable angina Angina that involves increasing pain and more frequent episodes that respond less and less to nitroglycerin or rest.

■ Cases

1. Your squad is dispatched to a retirement home where you find a 75-year-old woman reporting chest discomfort. Her caregiver tells you that the patient has been treated for angina for the last 3 years with limited problems. However, over the last several months, the frequency and severity of her angina attacks have increased. In addition, she felt no relief from three sprays of her sublingual nitroglycerin.

This information makes you suspect that this patient is at high risk for what event?

What other possibility exists relative to the patient getting no relief from her nitroglycerin?

2. A man in the checkout line at the grocery store collapses, prompting a call to 9-1-1. By the time you arrive on scene, the patient is conscious and seated on the floor, still in obvious distress. You apply a high concentration of oxygen, which improves the patient's color immediately.

What information should you attempt to obtain from the patient?

What other sources of patient information might be available for your assessment?

3. You are called to an extended care facility for a 67-year-old man having dizziness and shortness of breath. You arrive to find the patient in extreme distress in the care of nursing staff.

What are your immediate care priorities?

How might you obtain additional information if the patient cannot comfortably answer you due to the shortness of breath?

What items might you assess or reassess during the transport phase of patient contact?

CHAPTER 4

Rhythms of the Heart

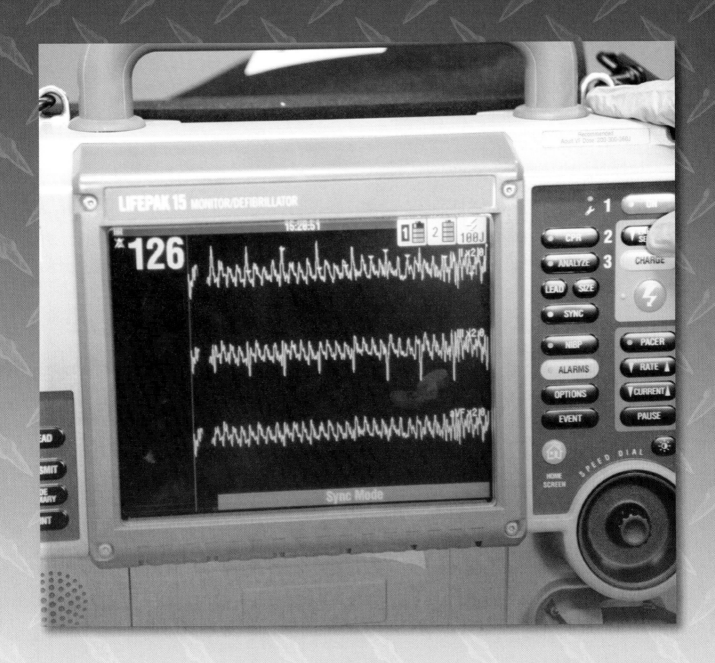

This chapter is designed to teach you how to recognize three ventricular dysrhythmias that are lethal if not treated immediately. The chapter focuses on teaching pattern recognition to enable you to quickly identify ventricular tachycardia (VT), ventricular fibrillation (VF), and asystole. The chapter also presents the treatments for each of the three dysrhythmias. You will also learn how to recognize electrical interference with your heart monitor and how to eliminate it.

The Pump of a Lifetime

The anatomic design and capabilities of the human heart are remarkable (**Figure 4-1**). The heart is a four-chambered pump that propels blood throughout the body. Each chamber is separated by valves that prevent the backwards movement of blood (**Figure 4-2**). There are even backup pacemaker sites should the primary pacemaker of the heart fail. These are all desirable features that allow the heart to meet the needs of continuous function from birth to death.

As with all muscle cells in the human body, the heart's cells have three properties that enable them to propel blood throughout the body. Each cell is able to respond to electrical stimuli, conduct electrical impulses, and contract (**Table 4-1**). The fourth property is unique to cardiac muscle cells and is called automaticity. Automaticity is defined as a cell's ability to initiate its own impulse. Groups of specialized cells form nodes in the heart that function as pacemakers. The primary pacemaker is called the **sinoatrial (SA) node** and is responsible for

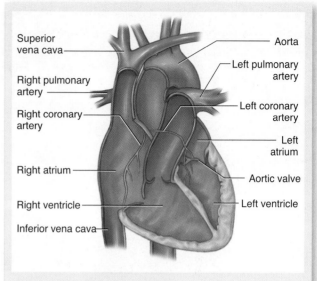

Figure 4-1   The human heart.

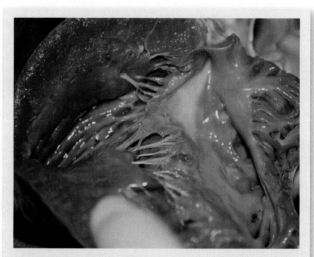

Figure 4-2   Heart valves.

Table 4-1   The Properties of Cardiac Muscle
■ **Automaticity**—The heart has the ability to initiate electrical impulses spontaneously without outside stimulation.
■ **Excitability**—The cells that make up the heart are able to respond to these electrical impulses.
■ **Conductivity**—These impulses travel through a type of internal wiring system throughout the heart.
■ **Contractility**—The cardiac muscle responds to electrical stimulation by contracting and pumping blood throughout the body.

triggering contraction of the heart 60 to 100 times per minute. Although the primary pacemaker of the heart is responsible for triggering contraction, it is ultimately regulated by the nervous and endocrine systems. For example, the parasympathetic nervous system is responsible for decreasing the firing rate of the primary pacemaker. Conversely, the sympathetic nervous system and endocrine system are responsible for increasing the rate. The atrioventricular (AV) junction is located at the bottom of the right atrium and can function as a backup pacemaker to the SA node. The AV junction has an inherent firing rate of 40 to 60 beats per minute. If the SA node ceases to function properly, the AV junction can take over pacemaking functions. Notice that the heart rate would then fall into the 40 to 60 beats/min range. Lastly, the ventricles can also function as the final pacemaker should both the SA and AV tissue stop working. The inherent firing rate of ventricular tissue is 20 to 40 beats/min (**Figure 4-3**). The conduction system is responsible for orchestrating the depolarization of heart cells in a very prescribed manner to ensure pumping efficiency.

When heart cells are at rest, the inside of the cells are negatively charged compared with the surrounding exterior and are said to be in a polarized state. Think of this polarized state as a state of readiness. When an electric current stimulates the cells, they electrically discharge and are said to have depolarized. The process of depolarization makes the muscle filaments contract and shortens the cell length, which is what makes the heart contract and pump. Repolarization is the process of returning all of the ions to their proper place in preparation for depolarization. The **electrocardiogram (ECG)** is a cardiac monitoring device that records all repolarization and depolarization activity on graph paper. Diseases can alter the flow of ions throughout the heart, resulting in a change on the graph.

With this basic understanding of cardiac physiology, you will now learn about the fundamentals of analyzing some of the key cardiac rhythms and the process of monitoring them.

▪ Rhythm Analysis

Assessing the Heart Rate

The quickest and simplest way to measure the heart rate is to count the number of QRS complexes that occur in a 6-second strip and then multiply that number by 10. The QRS complexes are the tallest or deepest waves on the ECG tracing (**Figure 4-4**). This method provides a close estimate of the heart rate per minute.

Now, you will learn how to determine the presence of VT, VF, and asystole on the ECG and how to treat each dysrhythmia.

▪ The Lethal Three

Ventricular fibrillation (VF), **ventricular tachycardia (VT)**, and **asystole** are cardiac rhythms considered to be lethal for good reason. Two of the three—VF and asystole—do not produce pulses, which means the patient is in cardiac arrest. The third—VT—is slightly more complex in that it may or may not produce a pulse. In the cases where VT is producing a pulse, it usually is not a rhythm that the heart can sustain for extended periods. At some point, maybe in 1 minute or in 30 minutes, VT usually deteriorates into VF, and the patient experiences cardiac arrest.

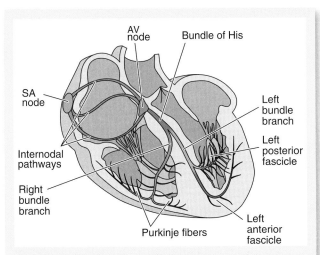

Figure 4-3 The electrical conduction system of the heart initiates an electrical impulse throughout the heart. The impulse travels through the cardiac conduction system and enables the four chambers to work together.

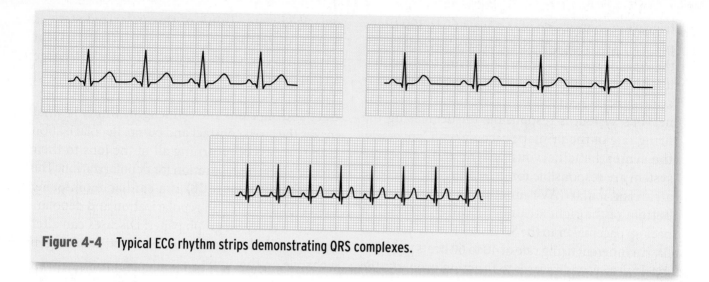

Figure 4-4   Typical ECG rhythm strips demonstrating QRS complexes.

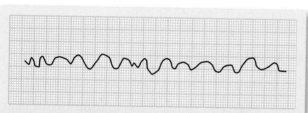

Figure 4-5   Ventricular fibrillation is a choppy disorganized rhythm.

In other cases, VT is the presenting rhythm but is pulseless. When this occurs, the condition is treated exactly like VF.

Ventricular Fibrillation

This is the most common presenting rhythm in sudden cardiac arrest, and when it occurs, the ventricles quiver rather than contract, resulting in no cardiac output and no pulse. When VF is noted, the patient should be assessed immediately to rule out muscle tremors, patient movement, loose lead artifact, or seizure activity.

If the rhythm is VF and the onset is recent, it will usually appear choppy (**Figure 4-5**). As time passes, the frequency and amplitude progressively decrease, producing what is termed fine VF. If left

untreated, VF will eventually degrade into asystole. The identifying features of VF are as follows:

- Heart rate cannot be determined
- Rhythm is grossly irregular
- No P waves
- No PR interval
- No QRS complex (replaced by choppy fibrillation waves)

Treatment

Once the patient is confirmed as pulseless and apneic, initial treatment depends on whether or not a defibrillator is available and on how long the patient had been in VF. If the arrest was witnessed and a defibrillator is available, it should be applied immediately, and the patient defibrillated. When a defibrillator is not available or if circulation has been disrupted for a period of time, chest compressions and ventilations should be administered.

Ventricular Tachycardia

Ventricular tachycardia (**Figure 4-6**) is a dangerous, unstable rhythm. Although it can produce a pulse, in many cases it does not. Given the fact that there is often preexisting heart disease often complicated by the current cardiac crisis, it is of little surprise that this

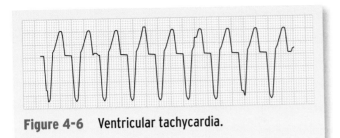

Figure 4-6 Ventricular tachycardia.

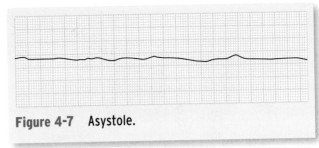

Figure 4-7 Asystole.

rhythm frequently deteriorates into VF within a few minutes. The identifying features of VT are as follows:

- Heart rate of 100 to 250 beats/min
- Regular rhythm
- QRS complex is wide, bizarre (greater than 0.12 seconds); often looks like large Vs side-by-side

Treatment

If the patient is alert with no signs of decreased cardiac output, the ALS team will insert an intravenous line and administer an antidysrhythmic medication, such as amiodarone, to terminate the dysrhythmia. If the patient is symptomatic with chest pain, decreased level of consciousness, hypotension, or cool, clammy skin, the preferred treatment for VT is the delivery of an electrical shock. Advanced providers may sedate patients prior to delivering electrical shocks to minimize the pain associated with the procedure.

Treatment for VT that does not produce any pulses (ie, pulseless ventricular tachycardia) is defibrillation.

Asystole

Whether it is called asystole, flat line, or cardiac standstill, this type of cardiac malfunction represents the complete cessation of electrical activity in the heart. When an adult patient presents in asystole, the prognosis is ominous. The identifying feature of asystole is the complete absence of electrical activity (**Figure 4-7**).

Treatment

The first phase of treating asystole is to confirm the presence of asystole in at least one additional lead. Chest compression should be administered immediately if the patient is unresponsive and has abnormal or absent breathing. In addition, a two-part check should be performed that includes the following:

- **Contact**—Make certain that the monitoring electrodes are securely attached to the skin by firmly pressing on them.
- **Connection**—Check that the patient cable is plugged securely into the cardiac monitor.

Treatment of asystole includes performing high-quality CPR, administering cardiac medications, and determining the reason behind the arrest and treating the causes. Patients that present in asystole have a very small chance of surviving.

TRAINING TIP

Have an in-service session where your ALS provider shows you how to properly connect the cables to the machine and patient. All rescuers must work together as a team during resuscitation efforts to maximize the patient's chance for survival.

Pulseless Electrical Activity

Pulseless electrical activity (PEA) is a condition where the ECG displays an organized rhythm but the patient does not have a corresponding pulse. PEA is not a rhythm but rather a condition. The causes of PEA can be remembered using the Hs and Ts. The Hs include hypoxia, hypovolemia, and hypothermia. The Ts include trauma, thrombosis (cardiac, pulmonary, brain), and toxins.

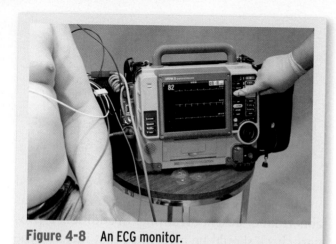

Figure 4-8   An ECG monitor.

Artifact

For a clean, easily readable ECG to be produced, various technical aspects of cardiac monitoring must be in place and working properly (**Figure 4-8**). If any of the following occur, the quality of the tracing may range from marginal to unreadable due to **artifact**, which in turn may contribute to less than optimal patient care (**Table 4-2**). Also, remember that leads need to be placed correctly in order to obtain a correct ECG reading (**Figure 4-9**).

Cardiac monitoring is a diagnostic procedure that provides important information about the overall function and stability of a patient's heart at a given moment. The ability to get the patient hooked

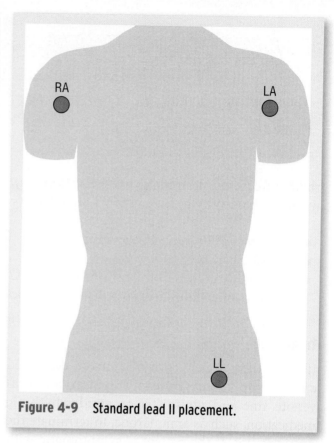

Figure 4-9   Standard lead II placement.

up quickly is another valuable function that the EMT can perform. In any case, cardiac monitoring is a key element of emergency cardiac care because lethal dysrhythmias are a common cause of death in these patients.

Table 4-2   Causes and Corrective Measures for Artifact

Causes/Condition	Corrective Actions
Poor electrode contact (wet or loose)	Dry any wet skin. If the electrode is loose, push it down firmly. Consider replacing the electrode.
Poor electrode contact (hairy skin)	Shave the chest area where the electrodes should be placed.
Loose lead	Snap the lead wire onto the back of the electrode.
Dry electrode	Replace the electrode with a new one.
Patient movement	Encourage the patient to be still.
Muscle tremor	If the patient is shivering, try to warm him or her. Confirm that seizure activity is not present.
60-cycle interference	Find the cause and unplug or shut it off. Common causes include heating pads, electric blankets, and microwave ovens.

PREP KIT

■ Vital Vocabulary

artifact Electrical interference that appears on the ECG that may mask or mimic the normal waveforms.

asystole A total absence of electrical activity on the ECG; also called flat line.

electrocardiogram (ECG) A tracing on graph paper that represents the electrical activity of the heart.

pulseless electrical activity (PEA) A condition where no pulse is felt on the patient despite having an organized rhythm on the ECG.

sinoatrial (SA) node A collection of specialized electrical cells located high in the upper right corner of the right atrium that serve as the primary pacemaker of the heart; also called the sinus node.

ventricular fibrillation (VF) A rhythm characterized by the absence of discernible waveforms on the ECG; a disorganized and chaotic appearing rhythm; the most common rhythm in sudden cardiac arrest.

ventricular tachycardia (VT) A rhythm characterized by wide complexes exceeding 120 beats/min on the ECG.

■ Cases

1. You arrive at the scene of a 56-year-old woman who reports crushing chest pain. Upon noting that she has a very slow heart rate and hypotension, you request an ALS ambulance. When the paramedics arrive, they place the patient on the cardiac monitor, which displays a sinus bradycardia at a rate of 44 beats/min.

   What is the correlation between this patient's bradycardia and her low blood pressure?

2. After assessing an elderly man as being unstable, you and your partner decide to arrange a rendezvous with an ALS ambulance because the closest hospital is approximately 30 miles away. When you meet the paramedics and begin assisting them with their care, you are asked to place the patient on a cardiac monitor. The ECG appears to indicate ventricular fibrillation, yet the patient is awake and talking.

   What is the most likely cause of the "ventricular fibrillation?"

   What would you do to troubleshoot the problem?

3. You are the EMT assisting a paramedic in the back of an ALS ambulance while transporting an unconscious patient to the hospital. IV therapy has already been initiated, and if the patient's SpO_2 is < 94%, oxygen is administered to maintain oxygen levels above 94%. The cardiac monitor is displaying a normal sinus rhythm at a rate of 80 beats/min. The paramedic asks you to palpate for a carotid pulse.

   What is the rationale for this request if the patient has a normal cardiac rhythm?

CHAPTER 5

Electrical Interventions in Cardiac Care

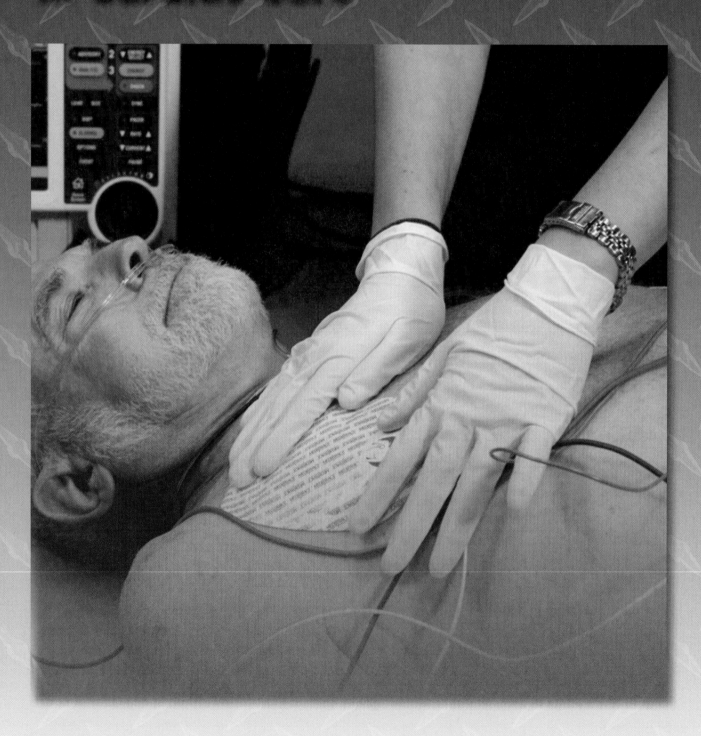

The human heart is an elegantly designed and efficient pump that constantly responds to electrical, chemical, and mechanical stimuli during its normal operation. In a stressed heart, this balance of stimulus and response is disrupted. Because the primary stimulus of the human heart is electricity, electrical interventions are used to manage some cases of cardiac dysfunction.

This chapter introduces you to the indications for the use of electrical interventions and explains the function and proper use of a defibrillator and external pacemaker.

■ Defibrillation

Aside from high-quality chest compressions, **defibrillation** is the treatment of choice for patients experiencing ventricular fibrillation (VF) or pulseless ventricular tachycardia (VT).

The concept behind defibrillation is simple: momentarily disrupt all electrical activity in the heart, terminating the lethal rhythm, and allowing the primary pacemaker to resume control.

> **TRAINING TIP**
>
> Familiarize yourself with the defibrillator used by your ALS response team. How much time have you spent in training for its use?

VF initially may be seen in 60% to 85% of patients in sudden cardiac arrest. When either VF or pulseless VT is present, the definitive treatment is defibrillation. Cardiopulmonary resuscitation (CPR) alone is less likely to terminate VF or pulseless VT. Performing continuous, uninterrupted CPR, however, is vital to keep the patient viable and to buy time until you can use the defibrillator. In these cases, CPR extends the window of time in which defibrillation may be effective (**Figure 5-1**).

> **TRAINING TIP**
>
> The chance for recovery of heart rhythm by use of defibrillation decreases by approximately 7% to 10% for each minute the heart continues to fibrillate, and even more so if chest compressions are interrupted.

The likelihood of surviving neurologically intact—having no brain damage as a result of cardiac arrest—is approximately 90% if the patient receives high-quality CPR and rapid defibrillation. When compared with the current survival statistics for all victims of out-of-hospital sudden cardiac arrest (4% to 5%), that percentage is remarkable. Defibrillation works best if it takes place as soon as possible after the dysrhythmia begins. Remember, to achieve better survival rates, seconds matter. Recurrent training and in-service practice will maximize your familiarity with the equipment and will minimize delays in delivering electrical therapy.

Intervention	Survival Rate
Early defibrillation (6 minutes) with CPR and ALS	30%
Early defibrillation (6 minutes) with CPR	20%
Delayed defibrillation (10 minutes) with CPR	2% to 8%
Delayed defibrillation (10 minutes)	0% to 2%

Figure 5-1 CPR is vital to extending the time in which defibrillation may be effective for patients in VF or VT, but CPR alone is unlikely to eliminate either rhythm.

Besides defibrillation, advanced cardiac care interventions may also include advanced airway management, pharmacologic therapy, and additional electrical interventions, such as cardiac pacing (discussed later in this chapter). Specific cardiac medication therapies will be discussed in the chapter, *The Fundamentals of Cardiac Pharmacology.*

■ Types of Defibrillators

Defibrillators are classified as either being manual or automated (**Figure 5-2**). The steps that must be performed by the operator vary with each type of defibrillator.

Manual Defibrillators

In most EMS systems, EMTs are not called on to perform manual defibrillation. However, as with other ACLS procedures, you may be called on to assist other providers with this skill. With manual defibrillation (**Table 5-1**), ALS providers must analyze the rhythm, determine the need to provide a shock and the appropriate energy setting, and depress the button.

Manual defibrillators typically are used by physicians, nurses, and paramedics because of the additional options and features offered, including the following:

- Synchronized cardioversion
- Cardiac pacing

Table 5-1   Manual Defibrillation With Hands-Free Pads
Steps
■ Confirm that the patient is unresponsive with abnormal breathing (apneic) and is in a shockable rhythm.
■ Turn the defibrillator on.
■ Select the energy level.
■ Place/apply adhesive hands-free defibrillation pads on the patient's chest.
■ Position the pads.
■ Charge the machine.
■ Clear the patient (visually/verbally).
■ Discharge the defibrillator.
■ Immediately resume chest compressions.

- Documentation options
- 12-lead ECG
- Waveform capnography
- Noninvasive BP monitoring
- ETCO$_2$ monitoring

With these options comes a need for the operator to not only be well versed in the operation and multiple functions of the machine, but also to be able to analyze and identify a wide variety of cardiac rhythms. Attaining this knowledge requires a comprehensive initial education and training as well as continuing education in order to maintain competency.

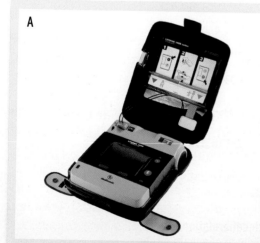
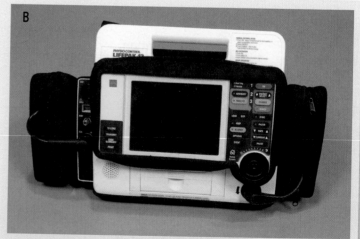

Figure 5-2   There are two types of defibrillators. **A.** Automated external defibrillator (AED). **B.** Manual.

Table 5-2	Automated Defibrillation

Steps

- Turn the defibrillator on.
- Apply the monitoring/defibrillation pads.
- Clear the patient (visually/verbally).
- Push the shock button if advised.

It is important to note that some manual devices also have a built-in AED feature, enabling BLS providers to use the devices prior to the arrival of ALS crews.

Automated Defibrillators

The steps necessary to operate the automated defibrillators are outlined in **Table 5-2**.

Safety During Defibrillation

One of the most hallowed rules of defibrillation is that the person pushing the button is ultimately responsible for safe operation of the defibrillator. Safe operation includes verifying that the patient is unresponsive and not breathing and that no one is touching the patient. Visually confirm that everyone is "clear" of the patient before delivering a shock. Immediately resume chest compressions following defibrillation.

■ Automated Implantable Cardiac Defibrillators

Automated implantable cardiac defibrillators (AICDs) (**Figure 5-3**) are devices implanted into patients who have experienced ventricular dysrhythmias. AICDs are designed to automatically detect lethal dysrhythmias and deliver an electrical counter-shock in an attempt to restore a normal cardiac rhythm.

Resuscitation measures should be initiated promptly in all cases where the patient is unresponsive and has abnormal or absent breathing, even if the patient has an AICD. If a cardiac monitor with a manual defibrillator is being used, hands-free monitoring/defibrillation pads should be placed on the patient's chest and the presenting rhythm identified. If the rhythm is shockable, then standard protocol

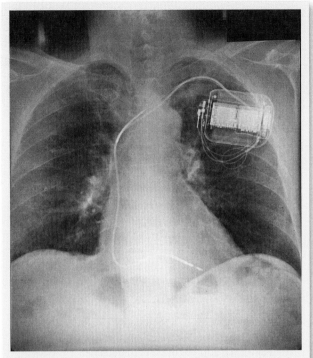

Figure 5-3 An automated implantable cardiac defibrillator (AICD) implanted into the chest.

and defibrillation procedures should be followed. If your unit has an AED, it should be applied and the protocol for its use followed.

EMT Interventions

With the continuing expansion of AED use, there is greater likelihood that you or possibly even a trained bystander may provide the initial defibrillation to the patient in cardiac arrest. Once the patient has been identified as being unresponsive and apneic, immediate initiation of CPR and rapid application of the AED are key components of patient care. Defibrillation, if indicated, should occur as quickly as possible. In addition, airway management using high-quality BLS techniques has been shown to improve patient outcome.

In some cases, you may have assumed care for the patient from citizen responders. In other cases, you may have initiated the primary care. Whatever the case, as long as the patient remains apneic and unresponsive, uninterrupted chest compressions should be performed.

AUTOMATED EXTERNAL DEFIBRILLATOR
Daily/Shift Inspection Checklist

Serial # _____   Date _____   Time _____

Model # _____   Inspected by _____

Item	Pass	Fail
Exterior/Cables		
Nothing stored on top of unit		
Carry case intact and clean		
Exterior/LCD screen clean and undamaged		
Cables/connectors clean and undamaged		
Cables securely attached to unit		
Batteries		
Unit charger is plugged in and operational (if applicable)		
Fully charged battery in unit		
Fully charged spare battery		
Spare battery charger plugged in and operational (if applicable)		
Valid expiration date on both batteries		
Supplies		
Two sets of electrodes		
Electrodes in sealed packages with valid expiration dates		
Razor		
Hand towel		
Alcohol wipes		
Memory/voice recording device—module, card, microcassette		
Manual override—module, key (if applicable)		
Printer paper (if applicable)		
Operation		
Unit self-test per manufacturer's recommendation/instructions		
Display (if applicable)		
Visual indicators		
Verbal prompts		
Printer (if applicable)		
Attach AED to simulator/tester:		
Recognizes shockable rhythm		
Charges to correct energy level within manufacturer's specifications		
Delivers charge		
Recognizes nonshockable rhythm		
Manual override system in working order (if applicable)		

Signature

Figure 5-4 Sample AED checklist.

■ Smooth Transition to ALS Care

Typically, when ALS crews arrive, they will want to switch to their monitor because of the additional capabilities it brings to patient care, eg, noninvasive blood pressure (NIBP), pulse oximetry, and waveform capnography.

If the defibrillation pads placed by the BLS crew are compatible with the ALS monitor/defibrillator, assist the ALS crew by connecting the pads to their device. Once the patient is hooked up to the ALS equipment, assist the ALS team with ventilations, deployment of a mechanical chest compression device, or preparing the patient for transport. Remember, it is critical to ensure high-quality chest compressions throughout the resuscitation attempt.

■ Defibrillator Care and Maintenance

Quite frequently, AEDs are the technology of choice for EMT squads because they are almost maintenance-free. Still, they are machines, and the possibility of mechanical failure, although small, exists.

Because of critical patient care implications in the event of an AED failure, each step should be taken to limit the likelihood of this occurring. One of the best ways to prevent AED failure is to follow the manufacturer's maintenance recommendations stringently, including the completion of any checklists provided to document any visual or physical checks to be routinely performed on the AED (**Figure 5-4**).

In the case of manual defibrillators, battery maintenance is one of the most important aspects of ensuring problem-free performance (**Figure 5-5**). Continued advances in battery technology have reduced the probability of battery failure. Be sure to follow the manufacturer's recommendations for battery care and optimization.

■ Synchronized Cardioversion

Synchronized cardioversion is the delivery of an electrical shock to the heart muscle at a very prescribed moment of the cardiac cycle. Synchronized cardioversion is used to treat patients experiencing rapid heart rates responsible for producing symptoms such as chest pain, low blood pressure, and altered mental status. Synchronized cardioversion is a skill reserved for ALS providers.

■ Transcutaneous Pacing

Transcutaneous pacemakers are used to manage slow heart rhythms. They are designed to detect the patient's underlying heart rhythm and stimulate contraction of the heart to maintain a constant rate of 60 to 100 beats per minute. Patients requiring transcutaneous (external) pacing often present with an altered level of consciousness. Once pacing is initiated, cardiac output is improved, and patients often regain consciousness and require sedation to manage pain associated with the procedure.

Internal or **implanted pacemakers** deliver very low doses of energy and pose no risk to the members of the EMS team (**Figure 5-6**).

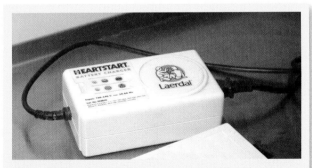

Figure 5-5 Battery maintenance is critical to an AED's performance.

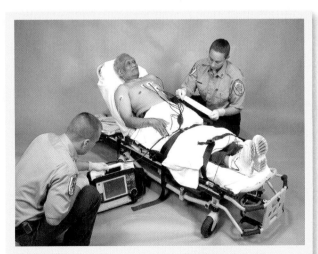

Figure 5-6 Patients may have implanted cardiac pacemakers. These pose no risk to emergency personnel and should not deter you from providing care.

PREP KIT

■ Vital Vocabulary

automated implantable cardiac defibrillator (AICD) A device inserted into a patient's chest designed to deliver an electrical shock if the heart experiences ventricular dysrhythmia.

defibrillation The act of simultaneously depolarizing the entire heart muscle with an electrical shock in order to allow a normal rhythm to resume.

implanted pacemaker A device that stimulates the heart to contract at a predetermined number of beats per minute.

synchronized cardioversion The act of simultaneously depolarizing the entire heart muscle with a timed electrical shock in order to restore a normal rhythm.

■ Cases

1. You and your partner are called to a residence for a man who cannot be awakened by his wife. When you arrive, you assess the man and find that he is pulseless and apneic. Your partner performs chest compressions as you attach the AED and initiate analysis of the patient's cardiac rhythm. It tells you that a "shock is advised."

   Why is it so important to deliver this shock immediately? By what percentage does this patient's chance for survival decrease if the shock is not delivered until 2 minutes later?

2. A 49-year-old man is complaining of pressure in his chest and nausea. After placing him on 100% oxygen, you begin to assess his vital signs. As you are taking his blood pressure, he suddenly loses consciousness. After determining that the patient is in cardiac arrest, you begin CPR as your partner attaches the AED.

   Assuming that this patient is in ventricular fibrillation, as are most patients with sudden cardiac arrest, why begin CPR if defibrillation is the most important therapy for this deadly rhythm?

3. Paramedics arrive on the scene where you and your partner are performing CPR on a man in cardiac arrest. Prior to ALS arrival, you delivered a shock with your AED, which has a screen that displays the patient's cardiac rhythm.

   Why might the paramedic ask you to bring your AED to the hospital?

CHAPTER 6

Fundamentals of Cardiac Pharmacology

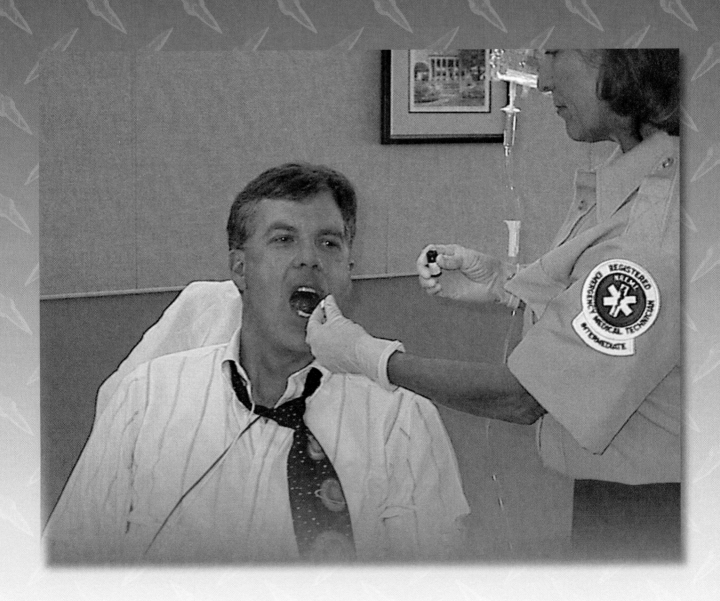

Chemical or drug intervention is frequently used in emergency cardiac care. This chapter presents an overview of the drugs most frequently used in sudden cardiac arrest and other cardiac cases. Each drug description includes its trade or generic name, its properties, and its desired effect on the body. After reading this chapter, you will have learned about to each drug's uses, effects, common dosages, and modes of delivery. As a result, you can positively affect patient outcomes as you work with ALS teams.

This chapter on **cardiac pharmacology** is intended to be a practical summary of the drugs used in emergency cardiac care to provide you with core knowledge regarding the following:

- Which drugs are commonly used in cardiac care
- The therapeutic benefits these drugs are intended to provide
- Which common side effects to stay alert for
- How each drug is usually administered
- The most common dosing regimen for each drug

Cardiac drug therapy is usually focused on addressing specific problems. Because of that, most cardiac drugs fall into distinct categories. In general, they either increase the heart rate, slow it down, make it less irritable, or make it more likely to respond to other therapies, such as defibrillation. Although some drugs have multiple functions, most are given for only one or two reasons.

Additional drugs discussed in this chapter are not necessarily specific to the heart, but are still used as therapies in cardiac care situations (**Figure 6-1**).

The EMT working in an ACLS environment requires only a basic knowledge of the drugs most commonly used to manage cardiac patients. Armed with this knowledge, you will know what positive effects to expect from certain drugs as well as what side effects to stay alert for when certain drugs are being administered by ALS personnel.

EMTs who have this increased knowledge of cardiac pharmacology will be an asset in the emergency situations they and the ALS teams face

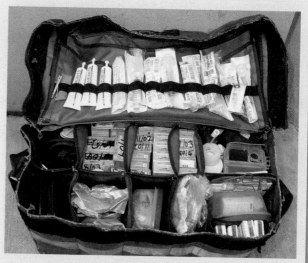

Figure 6-1   An ALS drug box.

every day. As most EMTs know, many prehospital cardiac calls often have to be managed by a single paramedic or ALS provider working in harmony with one or two BLS providers. This means that as ALS tasks are performed by the paramedic or ALS provider, many other aspects of call management and supervision must be assumed by the EMT or other BLS personnel.

The more trained and educated you are as an EMT working in the realm of ACLS, the better prepared you will be to anticipate the needs of your team and contribute to a positive outcome.

TRAINING TIP

After your next call with your ALS provider, find out the location of the primary drug box/jump kits. You will also want to know where to find the compartment where extra drugs are kept, for quick restocking when back-to-back calls keep the ambulance from returning to base for supplies.

■ The Language of Pharmacology

Pharmacology is a specialized branch of medicine. Some important words and phrases that you will need to be familiar with include the following:

- **Indications for use**—The reason(s) a certain drug is administered to a patient.

- **Contraindications for use**—The reason(s) a certain drug should not be administered to a patient.
- **Therapeutic effects**—The positive, or desirable, effect(s) expected to occur.
- **Side effects**—Predictable effects of a drug that are not part of the desired (ie, therapeutic) effect.
- **Allergies**—Sensitivity to a drug that results in an undesirable and potentially severe immune response with administration.
- **Half-life**—The amount of time it takes for half the drug to be metabolized and/or excreted by the body.
- **Dosage**—The amount of drug delivered to the patient. Dosage is most often stated in grams or portions of grams (eg, grams, milligrams, or micrograms) (**Figure 6-2**) because this denotes the actual weight of the drug. For each drug, there is a total allowable amount that can be given to a patient within a certain time frame, and this amount is typically weight-dependent. For example, 3 mg/kg of lidocaine is the maximum amount normally given in bolus form to an adult patient within any 1-hour time period.
- **Route of administration**—The method(s) by which a particular drug is given. Common routes include oral, inhalation, topical, and injection. In cardiac patients, most drugs are given intravenously (IV) because the drug reaches the heart more quickly. In the world of cardiac care, time is muscle—heart muscle, that is! You do not want a part of your patient's heart to die because a pill takes 45 minutes to dissolve in the stomach when the same drug could have been delivered to the heart through the bloodstream in seconds.
- **Inotropic**—Pertaining to the strength with which the heart contracts. If a drug is said to have a positive inotropic effect, it makes the heart beat stronger.
- **Chronotropic**—Pertaining to the rate or speed of the heart. If a drug has a positive chronotropic effect, it makes the heart rate speed up. A negative chronotrope does just the opposite: it slows the heart down.
- **Dromotropic**—Pertaining to the conduction of electricity. A positive dromotope will improve the conduction of electricity through the cardiac musculature.

Even though administration of almost all cardiac drugs is outside your scope of practice, this chapter will provide you with practical, baseline knowledge of the drugs most commonly used in emergency cardiac care, why and how they are administered, and what you should watch for after they have been given.

■ Common Cardiac Drugs

Oxygen

Because it is part of daily life, it is easy to forget that **oxygen** is actually a drug. When a person is breathing normally, atmospheric oxygen is inhaled 12 to 20 times each minute, but it is not considered to be a drug because oxygen exists naturally in the air. However, once oxygen is separated from the air into a pure substance and you place it in a green cylinder for a patient to inhale, it is considered a drug. Oxygen therapy can help prevent some of the most dangerous and undesirable abnormal heart rhythms.

Once the ALS team arrives, many patients are given epinephrine or vasopressin (to improve excitability), while others may receive lidocaine or

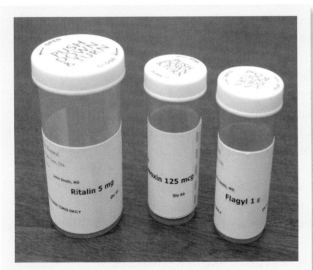

Figure 6-2 Dosage is usually stated in grams, milligrams, or micrograms.

amiodarone (to make the heart less irritable). Still others are given morphine or fentanyl (for pain management).

Patients may say that their heart feels "funny" or "different" or that their chest "aches." Those terms and others like them point to cardiac problems. Do not ever withhold oxygen therapy from any patient who is hypoxic. Titrate oxygen administration to maintain an Spo$_2$ of greater than 94%. Prophylactic administration of oxygen to all patients may not be helpful.

Nitroglycerin

Nitroglycerin is the most commonly used drug to treat patients with acute coronary syndrome (ACS). It has multiple uses, including the treatment of angina (exertional chest pain), heart attack, and heart failure.

Nitroglycerin is a potent, fast-acting drug. This smooth-muscle relaxant rapidly dilates peripheral and coronary vessels to decrease the workload of the heart and increase coronary blood flow.

Because of its potent **vasodilatory effects**, nitroglycerin can cause a patient's blood pressure to drop in a short time, especially in first time or infrequent users. You should obtain a baseline blood pressure before the patient is given the drug. In addition, remove all medication patches before administering multiple doses of nitroglycerin or other cardiac drugs.

Because nitroglycerin can cause a patient's blood pressure to drop quickly (in a worst-case scenario, causing a standing patient to fall), avoid this by making sure the patient is either lying down or seated safely when you administer the drug. Nitroglycerin is administered in the emergency setting either by a tablet under the tongue or by spray (**Figure 6-3**). Most patients get a moderate-to-pounding headache after receiving this medication, so be prepared to tell them that this is a normal and annoying, but not dangerous, side effect.

You should remember that many patients who have had chronic angina or a previous heart attack(s) may have their own supply of nitroglycerin and may have already placed one or two tablets under

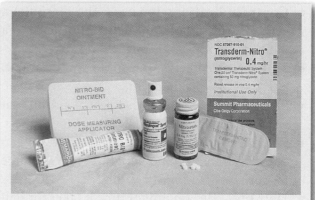

Figure 6-3 Nitroglycerin is one of the most commonly used drugs in cardiac care.

the tongue or administered several sprays (0.4 mg/ spray). Also, some patients wear nitroglycerin (nitro) patches that provide a timed release of the medication. Be careful when you are removing the patches. Wipe off any medication that gets on your skin, or you will have a pounding headache too.

Epinephrine

Epinephrine (**Figure 6-4**) is the name for the laboratory-created version of the hormone adrenaline. Adrenaline is made naturally by the body. It has many functions in survival, the most commonly known as the fight-or-flight response. Most people can recall feeling a surge of adrenaline when they barely escaped hitting another car while driving. There is a surge of energy to the major muscles, the heart, and the brain. It is this same immediate, powerful response that makes epinephrine so useful in cardiac medicine. This is especially true in sudden cardiac arrest management. The therapeutic effects of epinephrine include the following:

- Increased blood pressure
- Improved blood flow to the heart and brain
- Increased strength of cardiac contractions (when the heart is functionally pumping)
- Increased likelihood of successful defibrillation
- Improved ability for the heart to initiate an impulse (increased excitability)

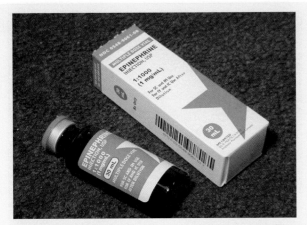

Figure 6-4 Epinephrine.

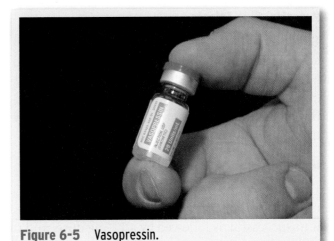

Figure 6-5 Vasopressin.

Because of its systemic **vasoconstrictive effects**, an important benefit of epinephrine is improved perfusion of the heart and brain. Epinephrine is also used for a variety of cardiac arrest rhythms. Under these circumstances, it is given every 3 to 5 minutes to increase excitability and responsiveness to defibrillation, with no dose limit as long as the patient is still pulseless and apneic.

Potential Side Effects

Side effects of epinephrine include significant increases in blood pressure and heart rate. You should frequently reassess vital signs to quickly recognize if the patient's condition deteriorates.

Vasopressin

Vasopressin (**Figure 6-5**) is a hormone that occurs naturally in the body, functioning primarily as an antidiuretic. In large doses, it becomes a potent vasoconstrictor that behaves much like epinephrine. Its use has gained favor because it does not seem to increase cardiac ischemia or irritability that may occur with epinephrine. Expect to see this drug used in a cardiac arrest when ventricular fibrillation or asystole is the problem. Vasopressin is usually given only one time during a resuscitation, although local protocols may call for a different dosing scheme.

Adenosine

Like epinephrine, **adenosine** (**Figure 6-6**) also is a naturally occurring substance produced in the

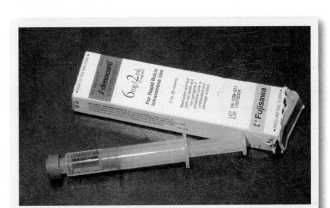

Figure 6-6 A box of adenosine.

body. The main therapeutic effects of adenosine are that it slows conduction through the middle of the heart (the AV node) and it can terminate fast rhythms in the AV node. One of the unique and challenging aspects of this drug is that once it is injected, the half-life of the drug is a matter of a few seconds! To get adenosine to the heart quickly, the drug is given first, and then followed immediately by a 10- to 20-mL saline push.

Another important feature of adenosine is that when it is exerting its beneficial effect, there is often a period in which the heart goes into asystole. When this occurs, expect a period of asystole ranging from 8 to 12 seconds or maybe longer. This can be unnerving for you when you watch a patient who just had a fast heart rate change to a phase where nothing but a straight line is seen on the cardiac monitor.

Potential Side Effects

Because of its unique and fast mechanism of action, side effects with adenosine are common and include flushing, dyspnea, and, occasionally, chest pain. Given the rapid action and short half-life of the drug, most of the side effects go away quickly.

Usual Dosage

Do not expect to see more than three doses of adenosine given to a patient. The initial 6-mg drug dose, if unsuccessful, is followed by a 12-mg dose, and if still unsuccessful, another 12-mg dose. Remember, a 10- to 20-mL saline flush follows immediately after each dose is given.

Lidocaine

Lidocaine works primarily on the ventricles. Dentists use this synthetic anesthetic to numb the pain caused by drilling into still living, innervated teeth.

The main therapeutic effect of lidocaine is to raise the fibrillation threshold of the heart and, therefore, it can help terminate and prevent repeat episodes of ventricular fibrillation (VF), although there is little in the literature to support its widespread use. Unfortunately, lidocaine usually does not help patients in VF who do not respond to defibrillation.

Lidocaine may be used as one of the drugs when the ventricles begin to produce ectopic beats on their own. It may also be used for cardiac arrest patients who present in either VF or pulseless ventricular tachycardia (VT). (As pointed out in the chapter, *Electrical Interventions in Cardiac Care*, although VF and pulseless VT are different cardiac rhythms, they are treated with the same approach, whether that is electrical or chemical interventions.)

Lidocaine comes packaged in two separate concentrations (**Figure 6-7**). The 2% preparation is intended to be injected into the IV line as a single dose and is not mixed. An infusion also exists and can be administered to patients to maintain constant levels of the drug in the blood. Although the packaging is clearly marked, it is good to understand the different doses and how they are administered.

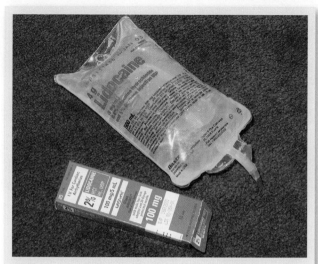

Figure 6-7 Premixed lidocaine used as a maintenance drip.

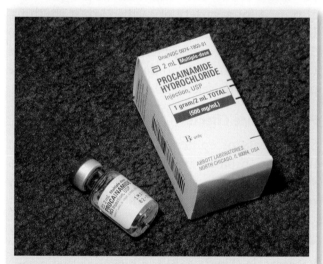

Figure 6-8 A multi-use vial of procainamide.

Procainamide

Procainamide (**Figure 6-8**) is comparable in its actions to lidocaine and is used in similar situations. However, unlike lidocaine, procainamide must be administered very slowly. Given the urgency of many cardiac emergencies, it makes sense that a drug that takes 5 or more minutes to administer would not be your first choice.

Expect procainamide to be used mainly for patients in VF or pulseless VT. When this drug is given to patients who have a pulse, procainamide has a potent vasodilatory effect in addition to decreasing the strength of the heart's contractions, so a falling blood pressure and hypotension are the most common side effects. Careful monitoring of the blood pressure is indicated, and you can assist with this. Lastly, procainamide also slows conduction of electricity through the heart.

Amiodarone

This antidysrhythmic drug is used in emergency cardiac care, primarily in the setting of persistent or recurrent VF or pulseless VT. Expect to see one to two doses of **amiodarone** (**Figure 6-9**) given during the treatment of sudden cardiac arrest when the heart does not respond to multiple shocks. Amiodarone is usually given either as a 150- or 300-mg dose.

Atropine

The main therapeutic effect of **atropine** is to increase the rate at which the heart paces itself by blocking parasympathetic stimulation to the sinoatrial (SA) node, the primary pacemaker of the heart (**Figure 6-10**). It also improves conduction (positive dromotrope) through the tissue in the middle of the heart located between the atria and ventricles, also known as the atrioventricular (AV) node.

Expect to see atropine used for patients with symptomatic bradycardia (a pulse rate of less than 60 beats/min with hypotension) or conduction problems, such as heart blocks.

A heart block is a condition in which an electrical impulse generated by the primary pacemaker of the heart, the SA node, fails to conduct down through the atria to the ventricles. For each of these blocked impulses that then result in "lost" contractions, a drop in blood pressure occurs. If enough of these impulses are blocked, blood pressure can drop significantly, causing the patient to experience loss of consciousness or to experience cardiac arrest.

Dosage

Atropine is a potent drug given in several small doses, usually 0.5 mg or 1.0 mg up to a total of 3 mg.

Potential Side Effects

Side effects of atropine include skin flushing, dry mucous membranes, delirium, and vision disturbances.

Magnesium

Magnesium (**Figure 6-11**) is a naturally occurring electrolyte found in the body. When the body has inadequate magnesium levels, it is common to see a high frequency of undesirable cardiac rhythms and possibly even cardiac arrest. For patients in VF, low levels of magnesium (hypomagnesemia) can cause the heart to become unresponsive, or

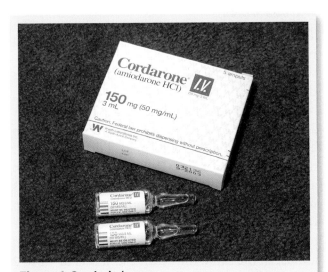

Figure 6-9   Amiodarone.

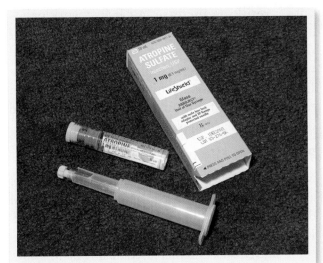

Figure 6-10   A box of preload atropine.

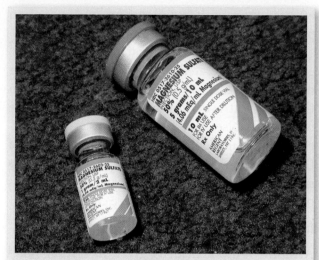

Figure 6-11   Magnesium.

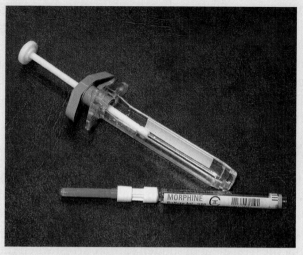

Figure 6-12   Morphine.

refractory (resistant), to conventional therapies. IV administration of magnesium reduces the frequency of complications for patients experiencing a heart attack. It also seems to keep patients from experiencing VT or VF and, as such, reduces the likelihood of sudden cardiac arrest. Magnesium is also used in the treatment of an unusual form of VT called **torsades de pointes**.

Morphine

Chest pain and increased anxiety are common signs and symptoms in cardiac patients. Collectively, they push patients further into the fight-or-flight mode with a resulting increase in cardiac workload—an undesirable situation for a malfunctioning or damaged heart. **Morphine** can be administered to patients with chest pain in certain situations. In some cases however, morphine has been shown to increase mortality in patients with acute and ongoing myocardial ischemia (**Figure 6-12**).

Potential Side Effects

Morphine is in a class of drugs called narcotic analgesics that cause central nervous system (CNS) depression, and, with that, respiratory depression. Respiratory depression is one of the most worrisome side effects, and increased dosing brings slow, shallow breathing. It is important to be alert for hypotension and the possibility of central nervous system depression, nausea, and vomiting.

Dosage

Because of CNS depression, expect to see morphine given in multiple small doses, usually 2 to 5 mg each. The maximum dosage allowed depends on local protocol. If too much morphine is administered and the patient becomes overly hypotensive, naloxone (Narcan) can be given in a dosage of 0.4 to 2.0 mg to reverse the effects instantly. Although this quick turnaround reverses the hypotension, expect the anxiety and chest pain to come back as well.

Nitrous Oxide

The use of nitrous oxide to control pain and anxiety in the cardiac patient is unique when compared with most other drugs discussed here because this drug is self-administered.

Nitrous oxide is an inhaled gas that is usually administered in a 50/50 concentration of oxygen and nitrous oxide. Patients hold the mask to their face and breathe in, usually receiving pain relief in about 1 to 2 minutes. If too much nitrous oxide is inhaled, patients quickly become drowsy and drop the mask, causing the effects of the nitrous oxide to quickly wear off. However, the nitrous wears off almost in the same time frame as it sets in—1 to 2 minutes—at which point, the patient reapplies the mask and begins breathing the nitrous oxide again, restarting the cycle of pain relief.

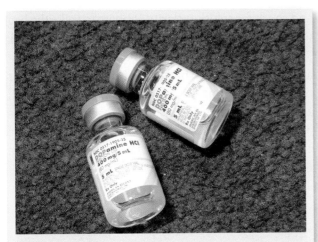

Figure 6-13 Dopamine.

Dopamine

One of the most unique agents found in the cardiac care drug box is **dopamine** (**Figure 6-13**). This selective inotropic agent/vasopressor is most commonly used to raise a patient's blood pressure.

Dosage and Delivery

Dopamine is usually added to a bag of IV fluid and administered by IV piggyback, allowing for continuous administration of the drug in the dose range indicated by the patient's condition.

Important Note

The effects of dopamine on the cardiovascular system are dose-dependent, which means that its effects are markedly different at different doses.

When given at low doses, (2 to 5 mcg/kg/min) dopamine improves blood flow to the brain, kidneys, and the mesentery. As the dosage is increased (5 to 10 mcg/kg/min), dopamine increases the heart rate. At dosages of 10 to 20 mcg/kg/min, dopamine causes peripheral vasoconstriction. Although this provides a quick marked improvement in blood pressure, the kidneys are adversely affected and potentially damaged, depending on the length of time dopamine has to be used.

As with some other drugs, dopamine increases the workload of the heart. However, the need to maintain adequate perfusion pressure takes precedence in this situation.

Indications

Expect to see dopamine used mainly for patients in cardiogenic shock, a life-threatening cardiac situation. A possible indicator of cardiogenic shock is an elevated heart rate, usually greater than 110 or 120 beats/min, and a low blood pressure, with a systolic blood pressure in the 60 mm Hg range or lower. When this mismatch of heart rate and blood pressure occurs in the context of a heart attack, cardiogenic shock is often the cause.

When a patient's blood pressure needs to be raised, the treatment choices include adding fluids and constricting the blood vessels. You can help by keeping a close watch on lung sounds that may indicate fluid overload.

> **TRAINING TIP**
>
> Ask your ALS provider agency to save the drug boxes after the next code in order to familiarize yourself with what they look like. This will make them easier to locate if you are asked to assist with a particular drug.

■ Intravenous Therapy

When intravenous (IV) therapy is being used, teamwork between BLS and ALS providers is critical. Given the time-sensitive nature of cardiac calls, your role in helping the patient receive IV therapy as quickly and smoothly as possible could contribute to making the call a success. Now that you have learned about various cardiac drugs, you will learn the steps for preparing a patient for IV therapy.

Choosing an IV Solution

In the prehospital setting, the choice of IV solution is usually limited to the **isotonic crystalloids** including normal saline and on occasion, lactated Ringer's solution. D_5W (5% dextrose in water) may also be administered, but is often reserved for administering medication because the presence of dextrose has the potential to alter fluid and electrolyte levels in the body.

Each IV solution bag is wrapped in a protective plastic bag, keeping it sterile until the posted expiration date. Once the protective wrap is torn and removed, the IV solution has a shelf life of 24 hours. The bottom of each IV bag has two ports: an injection port for medication, and an **access port** for connecting the administration set. The sterile access port is protected by a removable cover that represents a point-of-no-return line—once this cover is removed, the bag must be used immediately or discarded. It cannot be placed back in the drug box.

IV solution bags come in different fluid volumes (**Figure 6-14**). Volumes commonly used in hospitals are 1,000 mL, 500 mL, 250 mL, and 100 mL; the more common prehospital volumes are 1,000 mL, 500 mL, and 250 mL.

Choosing an Administration Set

An **administration set** allows the fluid to move from the IV bag into the patient's vascular system. As with IV solution bags, IV administration sets are sterile as long as they remain in their protective packaging. Once they are removed from the packaging, they must be either used or discarded. Each IV administration set has a **piercing spike** protected by a plastic cover. Once the piercing spike is exposed and the seal surrounding the cap is broken, the set must be used immediately or discarded.

There are different sizes of administration sets for different situations and patients. **Drip sets** have a number visible on the package (**Figure 6-15**), which indicates the number of drops it takes for a milliliter of fluid to pass through the orifice and into the **drip chamber**. Drip sets come in two primary sizes: microdrip and macrodrip. **Microdrip sets** allow 60 gtt (drops)/mL through the small, needlelike orifice inside the drip chamber. Microdrips are ideal for medication administration or pediatric fluid delivery because it is easy to control their fluid flow. **Macrodrip sets** allow 10 to 15 gtt/mL through a large opening between the piercing spike and the drip chamber. Macrodrip sets are best used for rapid fluid replacement (as is commonly required with trauma management) but can also be used for maintenance and **keep-the-vein-open (KVO) IV set-ups**.

Preparing an Administration Set

After choosing the IV administration set and the IV solution bag, verify the expiration date of the solution and check for solution clarity. Prepare to spike the bag with the administration set as indicated in **Skill Drill 6-1**.

Most, if not all, cardiac patients will need IV access should they have an immediate need for medications. Your efforts to help quickly establish a patent IV line will positively impact the outcome of the call, because the sooner the line is in place and functioning, the sooner the patient can get the medications needed.

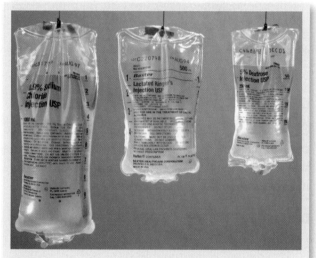

Figure 6-14   Examples of different IV bag sizes.

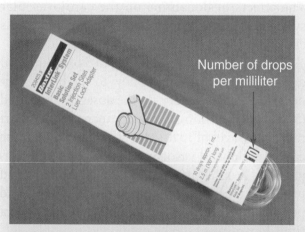

Figure 6-15   The number visible on the drip set refers to the number of drops it takes for a milliliter of fluid to pass through the orifice and into the drip chamber.

SKILL DRILL 6-1 Spiking the Bag

Remove the rubber cover found on the end of the IV bag by pulling on it. The bag is still sealed and will not leak until the piercing spike of the IV punctures this port.

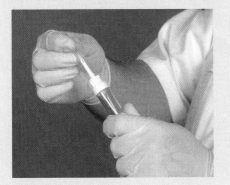

1 Remove the protective cover from the piercing spike (Remember, this spike is sterile!).

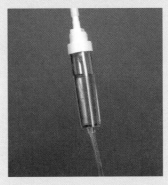

2 Slide the spike into the IV bag port and gently squeeze the drip chamber once or twice until it is half full.

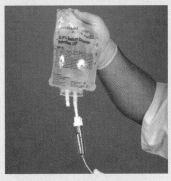

3 Allow the solution to run freely through the drip chamber and into the tubing to prime the line and flush the air out of the tubing.

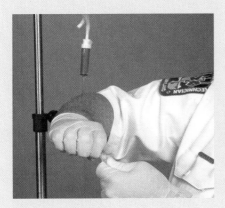

4 Twist the protective cover on the opposite end of the IV tubing to allow air to escape. Do not remove this cover yet, because the cover keeps the tubing end sterile until it is needed. Let the fluid flow until air bubbles are removed from the line before turning the roller clamp wheel to stop the flow.

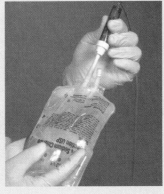

5 Next, go back and check the drip chamber; it should be only half filled. The fluid level must be visible to calculate drip rates. If the fluid level is too low, squeeze the chamber until it fills; if the chamber is too full, invert the bag and the chamber and squeeze the chamber to force some fluid back into the bag.

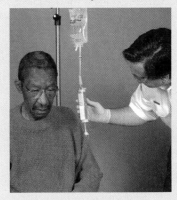

6 Hang the bag in an appropriate location with the end of the IV tubing easily accessible.

PREP KIT

■ Vital Vocabulary

access port A sealed hub on an administration set designed for sterile access to the fluid.

adenosine A naturally occurring substance produced in the body; also used as a drug in cardiac medicine to slow automaticity and conduction through the middle of the heart. Primarily used to treat regular, narrow complex tachycardias.

administration set Tubing that connects to the IV bag access port and the catheter in order to deliver the IV fluid.

amiodarone An anti-dysrhythmic drug given during sudden cardiac arrest when the heart does not respond to multiple shocks.

atropine A drug that increases the rate at which the heart paces itself by blocking parasympathetic stimulation to the sinoatrial (SA) node. This drug is used for patients with symptomatic bradycardias or other conduction problems.

cardiac pharmacology The study of drugs used in cardiac care and their therapeutic benefits, side effects, and administration.

dopamine An inotropic drug most commonly used to raise a patient's blood pressure in cardiogenic shock, usually administered by IV piggyback, and whose effects are dose-dependent.

drip chamber The area of the administration set where fluid accumulates so that the tubing remains filled with fluid.

drip set Another name for an administration set.

epinephrine A substance produced by the body (commonly called adrenaline), and a drug produced by pharmaceutical companies that increases the heart rate and blood pressure.

isotonic crystalloids The main type of fluid used in the prehospital setting for fluid replacement because of its ability to support blood pressure by remaining within the vascular compartment.

keep-the-vein-open (KVO) IV set-up A phrase that refers to the flow rate of a maintenance IV line established for prophylactic access, usually run in the 25- to 50-mL/h range.

lidocaine An anti-dysrhythmic drug used to raise the fibrillation threshold of the heart and prevent repeat episodes of ventricular fibrillation.

macrodrip set An administration set named for the large orifice between the piercing spike and the drip chamber. A macrodrip set allows for rapid fluid flow into the vascular system.

magnesium A naturally occurring electrolyte in the body; as a drug, it depresses the central nervous system, which may be useful in managing some cases of ventricular fibrillation in which the patient is resistant to conventional therapies.

microdrip set An administration set named for the small orifice between the piercing spike and the drip chamber. A microdrip set allows for carefully controlled fluid flow and is ideally suited for medication administration.

morphine An analgesic drug of choice when rapid anxiety and pain management are desired.

nitroglycerin Medication that increases cardiac blood flow by causing arteries to dilate; the EMT may be allowed to help the patient self-administer the medication.

oxygen A gas that cells need in order to metabolize glucose into energy.

piercing spike The hard, sharpened plastic spike on the end of the administration set designed to pierce the sterile membrane of the IV bag.

procainamide A drug similar in its actions to lidocaine, but that must be administered very slowly, thereby not making it the drug of first choice in cardiac medicine.

torsades de pointes An undulating sinusoidal rhythm in which the axis of the QRS

PREP KIT

complexes changes from positive to negative and back in a haphazard fashion.

vasoconstrictive effect The narrowing of a blood vessel, especially veins and arterioles of the skin.

vasodilatory effect The widening of a blood vessel.

vasopressin A hormone that occurs naturally in the body, functioning primarily as an antidiuretic. It becomes a potent vasoconstrictor when given in large doses.

■ Cases

1. A middle-aged man reports severe chest pain that radiates to his left arm and jaw. His blood pressure is 150/90 mm Hg, and his heart rate is 110 beats/min. You have just finished assisting the paramedic in initiating an intravenous line. Medical control has ordered the paramedic to administer morphine to this patient by the intravenous route.

   Why is it more beneficial to the patient to give this drug intravenously as opposed to direct injection into the muscle of the patient's upper arm? What potential side effects should you be alert for after the administration of this narcotic drug?

2. You request an ALS ambulance to respond to the scene of a patient reporting chest pain. Your rationale for this request was due to the fact that the patient's blood pressure was 70/40 mm Hg, and his heart rate was 140 beats/min. When the paramedics arrive, they assess the patient and decide to administer dopamine, which is an inotropic vasopressor drug.

   Through what effect will an inotropic drug raise this patient's blood pressure? Why would the paramedic not want to administer a positive chronotropic drug?

3. While you provide care to a 59-year-old woman with chest pain, she tells you that she took two of her prescribed nitroglycerin tablets prior to your arrival, but her pain has only improved minimally. You contact medical control and are advised to assist the patient with one more of her nitroglycerin tablets and then assess her blood pressure.

   What are the therapeutic effects of nitroglycerin in relieving chest pain of cardiac origin? What is medical control's rationale for asking you to obtain another blood pressure reading after administering the third nitroglycerin?

4. After performing defibrillation on a patient in cardiac arrest, the paramedic asks you to resume CPR. After establishing an intravenous line, epinephrine is administered.

   Through what effect(s) will this drug aim to enhance the effectiveness of the CPR that you are performing?

CHAPTER 7

Challenging Resuscitation Situations

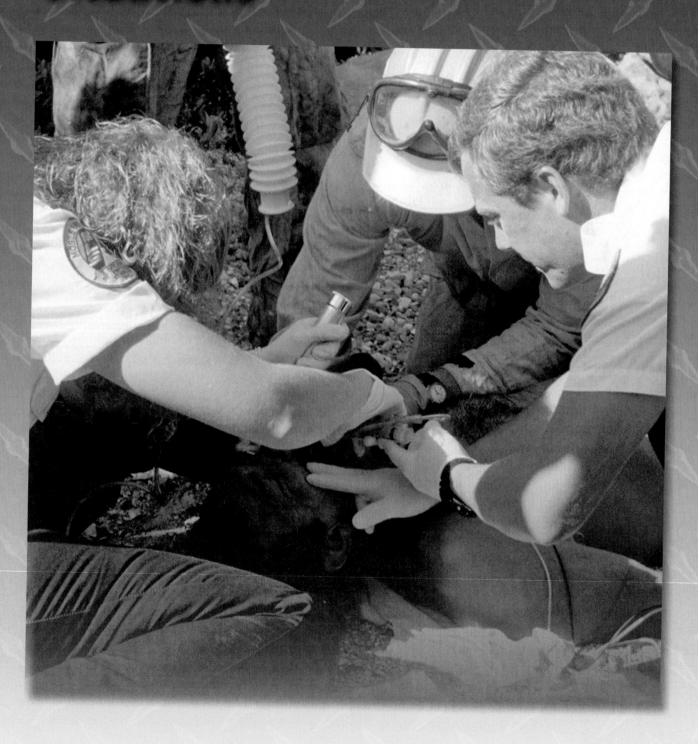

This chapter presents several of the most challenging resuscitation situations you will encounter, including stroke, electrical shock, lightning strikes, and large accident scenes. You will learn how to assess a stroke patient using the Cincinnati Stroke Scale. Drug-related cardiac emergencies are described, and the effects on patients produced by overdoses of both legal and illegal drugs are explained.

Few, if any, prehospital calls follow clinical or textbook presentations anywhere close to 100%. This chapter presents a number of challenging resuscitation situations that you may encounter, along with recommendations as to how you might best contribute to ALS patient care efforts.

■ Stroke or Brain Attacks

For years, **cerebrovascular accident (CVA)** was the term used to describe the condition resulting from decreased oxygen delivery to the brain, resulting in cerebral ischemia. In some cases, the CVA was caused by a blockage in a cerebral artery or reduction in blood flow, whereas in other cases, the culprit was a hemorrhage inside or around the brain itself. It is now known that this medical event is by no means an accident. To a great extent it is a predictable event and, to a lesser degree, a preventable one. As a result, this event is now called a stroke or brain attack.

In the past, a stroke patient was treated as a nonemergent patient, suggesting that the damage was present and irreversible. Because there was no hope of correcting the damage, there was little to be done other than to provide routine transport to the hospital emergency department (ED) to confirm the diagnosis and plan for the patient's long-term care. Recent advances in stroke treatment have caused a radical change in perceptions. Now, people know that if this often-catastrophic event is quickly recognized and treatment is started early enough after symptom onset, permanent damage can be avoided or reduced. This is especially encouraging news given the magnitude of the problem.

Stroke is the third leading cause of death in the United States in adults and is an important cause of long-term disability (**Table 7-1**). Approximately 500,000 Americans will have a stroke this year. For many, it will be a first-time occurrence. For others, it will be a recurrent event. Collectively, about 150,000 of these people will die. Given the absence of treatment options in the past, those who did survive often fared poorly from this profoundly life-changing event. Many were left unable to walk or communicate effectively, whereas others were left unable to even feed or provide basic care for themselves.

The use of fibrinolytics for the first time has offered medical practitioners a tool to reduce or reverse the neurologic insult frequently incurred by stroke patients. Research continues in the area of neuroprotective agents—another exciting and still emerging therapy. These agents may one day contribute to reducing mortality and morbidity even further.

As mentioned previously, the neurologic impairment resulting from a stroke is the result of two different mechanisms (**Figure 7-1**). **Ischemic strokes** result from the disruption of blood flow because of the partial or complete occlusion of a blood vessel supplying the brain. Roughly three out of four strokes are in this category, commonly as a result of blood clots that develop within a blood vessel in

Table 7-1 Top 10 Causes of Death in the United States in 2009

1. Heart disease
2. Cancer
3. Chronic, lower respiratory disease
4. Stroke
5. Unintentional injuries
6. Alzheimer disease
7. Diabetes
8. Influenza and pneumonia
9. Kidney disease
10. Suicide

Data Source: Centers for Disease Control and Prevention, Deaths and Mortality, http://www.cdc.gov/nchs/fastats/deaths.htm. Accessed 5/14/2012.

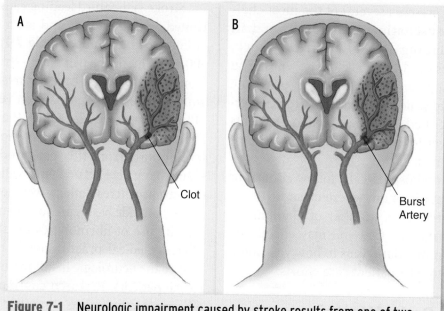

Figure 7-1   Neurologic impairment caused by stroke results from one of two different mechanisms: **A.** ischemic stroke, or **B.** hemorrhagic stroke.

the brain (<u>**cerebral thrombosis**</u>). The disruption also could result from clots that originated elsewhere in the body but moved through the cardiovascular system before finally causing a blockage in the brain (<u>**cerebral embolism**</u>). <u>**Hemorrhagic strokes**</u> are caused by disruption of blood flow as well, but in this case the precipitating event is the rupture of a cerebral artery, either above the surface of the brain or within the brain. Frequently, this event occurs as a byproduct of hypertension.

Currently, physicians have alternative methods of intra-arterial treatment of a patient experiencing an acute stroke. These options include use of "clot-busting" drugs, use of wires or balloons to dilate the occluded artery, and recently the use of specific "clot-retrieval systems" that pull or retract the clot from the vessel. A combination of any or all of these methods may be required to re-establish blood flow through the occluded artery. As mentioned earlier, patients experiencing an acute stroke are no longer considered to be "hopeless." Acute stroke patients must receive rapid assessment, aggressive treatment, and immediate transfer to definitive care. Acute stroke patients must be treated in systems of care with similar urgency as patients experiencing

heart attacks. You should think of an acute stroke as a "brain attack."

■ Risk Factors for Stroke

The most effective and certainly least costly approach to stroke is prevention, rather than trying to correct or repair the damage produced by a stroke.

Although some strokes occur without symptoms or warning, it usually is the exception rather than the rule. The predictors, or what might better be termed risk factors, for stroke have been identified and categorized as being either controllable or uncontrollable (**Table 7-2**). Those that are classified as controllable should either be eliminated or treated as much as possible, although genetics plays a role in these factors to some extent. By comparison, nothing can be done to diminish uncontrollable risk factors.

■ The Events Leading Up to a Stroke

Most strokes do not occur without warning. They are preceded by a series of <u>**transient ischemic attacks (TIAs)**</u>. A TIA is a neurologic deficit resulting from brain ischemia whose symptoms resolve within 24 hours. You can play a key role if the signs and

Table 7-2 Risk Factors for Stroke

Controllable Risk Factors
- Hypertension
- Heart disease
- Elevated cholesterol levels
- Diabetes
- Tobacco use
- Alcohol use
- Obesity
- Inactive lifestyle

Uncontrollable Risk Factors
- Age > 55 years
- Male gender
- Race
- Heredity
- Previous stroke

symptoms of a TIA are recognized. However, these signs and symptoms can be subtle and transient, which increases the difficulty of prompt recognition. With more training and education, recognition and care of TIAs in the field setting will improve.

Studies have shown that **tissue plasminogen activator (tPA)** improves neurologic outcomes if given to patients with ischemic stroke within 3 hours of symptom onset. Ideally, when a stroke patient is recognized in the field, a call can be made to alert the ED so fibrinolytic therapy can be initiated on arrival at the hospital.

TRAINING TIP

Make arrangements to observe stroke patients at a local rehabilitation facility. You will be able to see the various ways strokes can cause damage. Contact your local or state EMS authority to see if you can obtain continuing education credit toward your recertification.

■ Prehospital Care of the Stroke Patient

The good news is that you can help stroke patients survive until they arrive at the hospital. Most of the initial prehospital care commonly required by stroke patients falls within the scope of practice of EMTs.

Airway obstruction can result from paralysis of the muscles of the face, throat, tongue, and mouth. If positioning alone is not effective in maintaining an open airway, use of an oropharyngeal airway or a nasopharyngeal airway may be indicated. Suction should be set up and ready to remove saliva or vomit to reduce the risk of aspiration.

In the event that a traumatic event, such as a fall or car crash, may have accompanied the stroke, measures to restrict spinal motion may be indicated. Whenever possible, place the patient in a neutral position, place a rigid cervical collar, and use care when log rolling the patient onto the backboard or when placing the patient in the recovery position.

Be alert for abnormal respiratory patterns such as Cheyne-Stokes or central neurogenic hyperventilation. Hypoventilation from shallow respirations or poor air exchange can also be a concern. You may gain even more valuable insights by using the Cincinnati Stroke Scale (**Table 7-3**). Stroke patients requiring rescue breathing for respiratory arrest secondary to their cerebral event should not be expected to have a positive outcome, irrespective of the patient care interventions provided.

Of course, some stroke patients require ALS interventions to supplement the initial BLS care. You can be helpful in making the call to request ALS. Advanced airway management techniques may be considered if BLS maneuvers are inadequate to sustain and protect the airway. Intubation can

Table 7-3 The Cincinnati Stroke Scale			
What to Look For	**How to Evaluate**	**Normal**	**Abnormal**
Facial droop	Ask the patient to smile or show you his or her teeth.	Face is symmetric and both sides move equally well.	Asymmetry and/or unequal facial movements.
Arm drift	Have the patient close his or her eyes and hold the arms out.	Both arms remain still or move the same.	One arm drifts down or does not move.
Speech	Ask the patient to say "You can't teach an old dog new tricks."	Patient uses correct words with no slurring.	Patient cannot speak, slurs words, or uses inappropriate words.

be performed by EMTs in some EMS systems. In systems where this is still not allowed, however, the EMT can assist the paramedic or other ALS provider during intubation.

In addition, cardiovascular complications are common in the context of stroke. There are some cases in which a cardiac condition may have caused the stroke, as in the case of blood clots forming as a result of atrial fibrillation. With this particular rhythm, the top two receiving chambers of the heart (the atria) fibrillate, or quiver uncontrollably, without producing effective pumping action. When this happens, the blood moves sporadically into the ventricles, occasionally sitting long enough for clots to start forming. There also is an estimated 25% drop in cardiac output when atrial fibrillation occurs. This cardiac rhythm is infrequently treated in the field setting unless the ventricular response is greater than 100 and produces hypotension and an unstable condition. When cardiac events are associated with a stroke, careful monitoring of the patient's blood pressure and cardiac rhythm is always a good idea.

Another ALS intervention indicated is intravenous (IV) access. A saline lock usually will suffice, because fluid resuscitation is rarely indicated for these patients, so the point of the IV access is for drug administration purposes. Drug therapy may be required for seizure control or treatment of hypoglycemia or dysrhythmia. If IV fluids are administered, isotonic fluids are the fluids of choice and should be run at either "to keep open" (TKO) rates or less than 30 mL/h, unless hypovolemia is identified as a problem.

■ Trauma-Induced Cardiac Arrest

Cardiac arrest that occurs secondary to trauma is a grave event associated with poor outcomes. The most common traumatic causes/mechanisms include:

- Airway obstruction
- Devastating head trauma
- Massive blood loss
- Great vessel damage
- Extensive damage directly to the heart

- Tension pneumothorax
- Cardiac tamponade

Given the extent and severity of body damage represented by these mechanisms, the dismal survival numbers come as no surprise. Poor survival, however, does not imply that you should give up and do nothing for the patient. To put this challenging situation in perspective, the following section describes how to work through the process.

When you are dispatched to a serious trauma scene or event as identified by the caller, a request for ALS should be made immediately (**Figure 7-2**). If a helicopter routinely transports seriously injured patients to a local trauma center, contact the center and put personnel on standby (**Figure 7-3**). This will allow the flight team to start the preflight routine, evaluate weather conditions, and identify the most appropriate landing zone near the emergency scene.

If patients have been determined to be in cardiac arrest prior to your arrival at the emergency scene, do not consider this an indisputable fact. An injured patient with extensive blood loss may have a very fast, weak pulse that was overlooked by the person who made the determination. The person may have also checked a radial pulse, which, given a number of severe injuries or condition, may not be present. In some cases, a carotid pulse may still be palpable but may not have been checked.

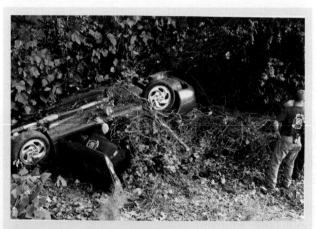

Figure 7-2   When dispatched to a serious trauma scene, request ALS immediately.

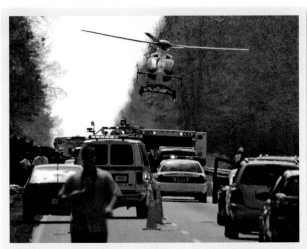

Figure 7-3 A helicopter may be used to transport patients quickly to a trauma center.

This could also lead to the erroneous assumption that the patient is in trauma-induced cardiac arrest. Do not take for granted that any patient is in cardiac arrest unless identified as such by an EMS professional.

Again, make certain that ALS is en route. If they have not already been requested, call them immediately. Keep in mind that it is better to request ALS and not need them than to have a patient suddenly deteriorate and need ALS interventions only to find out that ALS is not on scene, or worse yet, not en route.

Some of the common causes of trauma-induced cardiac arrest and the corresponding EMT interventions include those listed in **Table 7-4**.

For patients who are seen in cardiac arrest but do not have obvious signs of serious trauma, the cardiac event may have preceded the traumatic event. In this case, apply an automated external defibrillator (AED), if one is available. If the patient is in ventricular fibrillation (VF), rapid defibrillation may be successful. If the patient is in VF secondary to blood loss and the fluid and electrolyte imbalance that results, electrical therapy in the form of defibrillation will not solve the problem.

You should address any other conditions identified as being correctable or controllable, because these may result in a successful resuscitation or prevent cardiac arrest from occurring.

■ Hypothermia

Whenever a person's body temperature drops below 95°F, the condition is known as **hypothermia**. Hypothermia can occur suddenly—for example, by submersion in freezing water after a fall through ice. In a scenario such as this, the person can become mentally and physically incapacitated in just a few minutes. By comparison, an elderly person who falls to a cold tile floor, fractures a hip, and then lies there for several hours also can become hypothermic. Although these situations are distinctly different, each can produce a similar result.

Regardless of the mechanism, as the body's core temperature begins to fall, normal body functions begin to falter. A core temperature of 95°F to 86°F would be classified as mild hypothermia. Once the core temperature dips below 86°F, cardiac output falls, blood pressure drops, and blood flow to the brain decreases. This is classified as severe hypothermia. Because of the slowed metabolic state, a patient can appear to be clinically dead, but there is a possibility that resuscitation can be accomplished with little or no residual neurologic deficit. It is impossible to predict the outcome based on the initial patient presentation in the field setting.

Your initial assessment of pulse and respirations on a cold patient should take a full minute to obtain an accurate rate. If the patient is determined to be pulseless and apneic, CPR should be initiated. During any patient care/resuscitation situation in which hypothermia may be a factor, preventing further heat loss is also a major issue. As the patient's core temperature drops, the situation becomes more critical. Remove wet clothing and cover the patient with blankets, preferably warmed. Move the patient out of the cold environment and into a warm ambulance as soon as possible. If that is not possible in the short term, steps should be taken to shield the patient from the wind, rain, or other elements.

Make certain that ALS is en route because cardiac monitoring is one of the keys to keeping a handle on the patient's condition. IV access is also desirable. If ALS cannot be on scene quickly,

Table 7-4   Critical Trauma/Trauma Arrest

Mechanism/Indicators	EMT Actions
Devastating Head Trauma 1. Patient presents as unconscious and unresponsive during the initial assessment, then has cardiac arrest. 2. Obvious mortal head wound. Gray matter visible.	Assess and secure the airway, stabilize the spine, begin CPR, contact the base station for a decision to transport or to discontinue resuscitative efforts.
Massive Blood Loss 1. Large amount of visible blood on the patient/ground. 2. Unable to produce a pulse with CPR, even with increased depth of compressions.	Control bleeding and reassess the carotid pulse. If a pulse is present, request ALS or air medical transport. Keep the patient warm. Contact the base station.
Airway Obstruction 1. Patient presents in an anatomically incorrect position. 2. Poor patient color. 3. Unable to ventilate.	Open the airway and attempt to ventilate while maintaining spinal motion restrictions. If unsuccessful, reposition the jaw and attempt to ventilate again. Suction and insert the oropharyngeal or nasopharyngeal airway. Repeat until the obstruction is cleared.
Great Vessel Disruption 1. Poor patient color/pale. 2. Unable to produce a pulse even with increased depth of compressions.	Reassess the carotid pulse and control bleeding. Request ALS if not already done. If CPR has already been initiated, contact the base station for orders, possibly to discontinue resuscitative efforts.
Tension Pneumothorax 1. Anxious patient, decreased level of consciousness. 2. Extreme dyspnea. 3. Distended neck veins. 4. Weak, thready pulse (narrowed pulse pressure). 5. Absent breath sounds on one side. 6. Tracheal deviation (late sign, often associated with cardiac arrest).	Apply high-flow oxygen by nonrebreathing mask or assist ventilations with a bag-mask device. Request ALS, request air medical transport, or arrange for an ALS rendezvous. Perform needle decompression if authorized.
Cardiac Tamponade 1. Anxious patient, decreased level of consciousness. 2. Distended neck veins. 3. Weak, thready pulse. 4. Narrowed difference between systolic and diastolic numbers. 5. Muffled heart tones.	Request ALS or air medical transport. Contact the base station for orders. Consider immediate transport. Perform CPR if cardiac arrest occurs en route.

initiate transport immediately. A hospital offers far superior technology choices for active rewarming of a patient.

Handle hypothermic patients gently to minimize the chance of inducing VF in severely hypothermic patients. Even a procedure such as endotracheal intubation has been reported to cause VF in situations involving hypothermia. Field resuscitations are difficult enough without the added complications resulting from hypothermia, which makes it even harder still to resuscitate the patient successfully.

■ Electrical Injuries

Most of today's modern conveniences would not be possible without electricity. Although electricity has improved our quality of life, it causes harm when

When an electric current passes through the brain, it can precipitate respiratory arrest. A similar result can occur if the diaphragm and other respiratory muscles are paralyzed by the electric current. This condition can persist for several minutes after the patient has been removed from the electric source. You must be alert for these conditions. If respiratory arrest goes unrecognized and untreated for more than a minute or two, the progression of hypoxia to **anoxia** will result in a full arrest situation.

Whenever you are called to care for a possible electrical injury, remember that rescuer safety is your priority. Only when that has been addressed can patient care commence.

Because of the many variables involved with electrical injuries, rapid assessment and management are essential. This is true for all patients with electrical injury but even more so for younger patients who have little or no cardiovascular disease, which makes them easier to resuscitate. No matter what the age of the patient, you and the members of your team should aggressively resuscitate all patients with problems related to electricity exposure, even those who appear dead during the primary assessment.

All the pieces of EMT care need to fall quickly into place when you are caring for patients who have been exposed to electricity. Secure the airway, determine adequacy of breathing, and provide high-flow oxygen if appropriate. Initiate CPR if indicated. If the possibility of head or neck trauma is present, take precautions to restrict spinal motion. Extinguish smoldering clothes and remove them quickly, along with any watches or constricting jewelry that may worsen tissue damage. Apply an AED immediately if the patient is pulseless and apneic.

Another pivotal decision to make is to request ALS for these patients as soon as possible. The burns and fractures commonly associated with more severe electrical injuries can warrant IV fluid replacement to counter hypovolemia. Electrical injuries can produce swelling in and around the airway, which may need ALS interventions. Extensive drug therapy also may be required, depending on the damage to and the response of the heart and

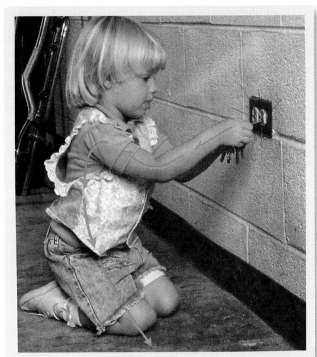

Figure 7-4 Electricity can be harmful if it enters the body.

it enters the body (**Figure 7-4**). Depending on the characteristics of the electrical source—for example, volts, amps, resistance, as well as the duration of the contact—the effect of exposure to electricity can range from a mild tingling sensation to cardiac arrest.

Electricity damages the body by the conversion of electric energy to heat energy as it passes through body tissues. Resistance plays a large factor as well. An intact skin surface is the most important factor impeding current flow into the body. Once the skin is cut or broken, it is far less effective in its protective qualities. The same is true (only to a lesser degree) if the skin is wet.

The voltage of the electric current also is an important factor, with high and low voltage each having unique characteristics. Low voltage follows the path of least resistance in and through the body, primarily through blood vessels, nerves, and muscle. In addition, low voltage (specifically alternating house current) is much more likely to produce VF, whereas contact with direct current is more likely to produce asystole. By comparison, high voltage takes the shortest distance to reach the ground.

cardiovascular system. In all cases involving electric shock, continuous cardiac monitoring is indicated because some cardiac rhythm disturbances that are initially absent may reappear as time passes.

Lightning-Related Injuries

Although lightning may well be one of the most impressive and magnificent natural phenomena, it is also the most deadly, killing up to 300 Americans each year (**Figure 7-5**). Almost double that amount will sustain serious injuries as a result of their exposure to lightning.

When compared with the seemingly minute amount of electricity represented by house current, it seems miraculous that a person could survive an encounter with 100 million to possibly 2 billion volts of electricity from a lightning bolt. In fact, only about one third of people hit by lightning end up dying from their injuries. The duration of exposure is only a fraction of a second, with almost all of the current "flashing" over and around the surface of the patient, which explains the high survival rate. However, the two thirds who survive will almost all have some form of long-term disability. A small

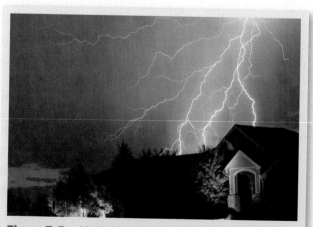

Figure 7-5   Lightning kills up to 300 Americans each year.

amount of the current from a lightning bolt can kill a person instantly. When this happens, the lightning strike can be thought of as a single, massive defibrillation that depolarizes the heart, usually resulting in asystole. Even if this primary cardiac event does not occur, damage to the respiratory center in the brain or the resultant paralysis of the muscles of respiration can leave the patient in respiratory arrest. As mentioned previously, if this condition is not identified and addressed immediately, it will quickly progress into full cardiac arrest.

Another unusual characteristic of lightning is that a single strike can injure or kill multiple people through what is often referred to as a **splash effect**. When this occurs and multiple patients are down, a principle called **reverse triage** is employed. In this case, the dead are actually treated first because they may be resuscitated with rescue breathing alone and cardiac arrest may be reversed.

Aside from this break from the traditional triage process, the remaining care is handled in the usual fashion. For those patients in respiratory arrest, rescue breathing with supplemental oxygen is indicated. Remember, if the respiratory arrest was precipitated by paralysis of the muscles of respiration, the patients may resume spontaneous respirations once they regain control of their musculature, allowing the rescue team to focus their resuscitative efforts on other patients.

Other therapies, such as CPR, the energy levels for defibrillation, drug sequencing, and drug dosing, all remain unchanged. Keep in mind that an unseen brain injury may have occurred, so stay alert for signs of an evolving head injury or rising intracranial pressure as indicated by changes in level of consciousness or vital signs.

Drug-Related Cardiac Emergencies

Illicit drug use of both naturally occurring and synthetic substances has been documented for hundreds of years. The Aztecs were reported to be habitual users of hallucinogens, particularly psilocybin mushrooms. Cocaine use was written about in the 6th century, and its use almost certainly predates that of the peoples of South America, where the coca plant is indigenous.

A drug-related emergency can be thought of as either travel down the high road or the low road in terms of the body's response. Travel down the high road involves the amphetamine and amphetamine-like drugs, which include both legal (licit) as well as illegal (illicit) substances. The legal agents can be divided further into prescription and over-the-counter products (**Figure 7-6**). By comparison, travel down the low road is usually brought about by heroin, other narcotics, designer analogs of narcotics, other central nervous system (CNS) depressants, or sedative hypnotics.

The High Road

Estimates regarding cocaine use place millions of Americans as regular users. In its natural state as coca leaves, the purity is only around 2%. Once processed into cocaine hydrochloride, product purity can approach 100%. The freebase form of cocaine, or "crack" cocaine, also has high levels of purity.

The toxicity of cocaine differs for each person, and depends on the combination of purity, dose size, and method of use. For example, powdered

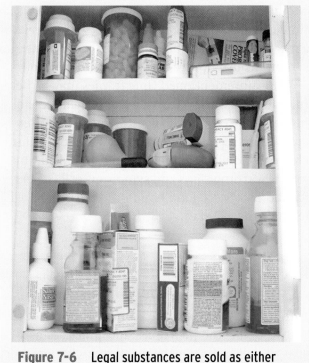

Figure 7-6 Legal substances are sold as either prescription or over-the-counter products.

cocaine that is sniffed may take several minutes to manifest its effects, whereas inhaling one "hit" of crack cocaine from a pipe can produce an even more intense physiologic response in less than 10 seconds.

A rapid rise in heart rate and blood pressure is common, as is chest pain, which is often what prompts a call to EMS. When cocaine is smoked, the strain on the heart, lungs, and brain is amplified, increasing the likelihood of stroke, seizure, or cardiac problems.

Possibly one of the most lethal reactions to cocaine use is decreased blood flow to the heart in combination with vasospasms that can close coronary arteries. This reaction can result in a myocardial infarction in a person who does not have blockage of a coronary artery.

For cocaine abusers with preexisting heart conditions, the body's response to cocaine can easily trigger a cardiac emergency and a call to 9-1-1. It is common for the symptoms resulting from cocaine use to resolve as the effects of the drug wear off, usually within 45 to 60 minutes. Nonetheless, the increased cardiac workload and increased oxygen consumption that accompanies it, coupled with chest pain and increased levels of anxiety and fear, may result in a call to EMS.

When you are confronted with a possible drug-induced cardiac emergency, you should request an ALS response. Should the patient have a cardiac arrest, VF is the most common presenting rhythm. Rapid defibrillation and excellent BLS code management are paramount to give the patient the best chance at survival.

Designer Drugs

There are many readily available drugs, both legal and illegal, related to cocaine and amphetamines in their chemical structure as well as in their effects. Many nasal decongestants and diet aids fall into this category.

Designer drugs are compounds that have been altered in a clandestine drug laboratory setting to make them more potent and/or to skirt existing drug laws. The passage of the Designer Drug Law in the early 1980s has helped to close the legal loophole that these clandestine chemists were using, but has done little to get these drugs off the street. Methamphetamine labs are among the most dangerous scenes any EMS provider may encounter for a variety of reasons, including toxic and flammable chemicals, carcinogenic by-products of the drug-making process, and gun-toting members of the drug trade.

Any drug that speeds up the heart also increases the heart's need for oxygen. As such, administration of high concentrations of oxygen and efforts to reduce patient anxiety are both EMT interventions that can be beneficial.

The Low Road

For the last few years, narcotics (specifically heroin) have been the primary drugs that have taken users down the low road to cardiac arrest. These drugs can be naturally occurring opioids such as opium and heroin, or the synthetic narcotics such as fentanyl or meperidine (Demerol). In either case, the drugs are all CNS depressants that may slow respirations to the point that the user becomes profoundly hypoxic. Again, when the heart's oxygen demands are not met, it becomes irritable, and a variety of cardiac rhythm disturbances appear. When slow heart rates result, expect the blood pressure to fall. Narcotics also cause vasodilation, which can further contribute to hypotension. Therefore, your careful monitoring of the blood pressure is a valuable contribution when you are caring for these patients.

The person who experiences cardiac arrest as a result of narcotic abuse may do so secondary to respiratory depression and/or respiratory arrest. Once again, the prevention of prehospital cardiac arrest is paramount. You or another EMT should provide assisted ventilations for patients who are breathing at fewer than 10 breaths/min or are mentating poorly. If the patient's SpO_2 is < 94%, oxygen should be administered to maintain oxygen levels above 94%. If respiratory arrest occurs, effective care by you and your team may prevent cardiac arrest.

The narcotic antagonist naloxone (Narcan) is used to reverse the CNS effects. If your service does not allow the use of naloxone by BLS providers, ALS providers will most certainly carry the medication.

In most cases, a single dose can instantly reverse the effects of the narcotic. This may not always be the case with some of the designer narcotics, such as 3-methyl fentanyl, which is between 3,000 and 5,000 times as potent as heroin.

Tricyclic Antidepressants

When taken in the prescribed dose, it is unusual for **tricyclic antidepressants (TCAs)** to produce serious side effects, and to their credit, they have helped countless people live normal lives. However, when taken in excessive quantities, either accidentally or in a suicide attempt, TCAs are some of the most **cardiotoxic** medications. When taken in conjunction with alcohol, their potential lethality rises even further.

In a potential TCA overdose situation, prompt ALS response is indicated. If that is not possible, immediate transport should be initiated, because these patients can decline quickly. In addition to maintaining a patient's SpO_2 level to above 94%, be alert for the signs and symptoms of developing TCA toxicity, which include increasing heart rate, seizures, decreasing level of consciousness, dilated pupils, and hypotension. Sudden respiratory arrest is also a possible occurrence in patients experiencing a TCA overdose. If a reasonably accurate time of ingestion can be identified, it can serve as a measurement tool, because most of the signs and symptoms usually are seen within 1½ to 2 hours.

The aforementioned time frames may be helpful, but only if they are accurate. When alcohol is involved with the TCA ingestion, which it often is, any patient-reported time frames should be considered questionable. Therefore, you should stay alert for the warning signs and symptoms of TCA toxicity and provide a good hand-off report to the ALS team or the ED staff.

■ Considerations with Pediatric and Neonatal Resuscitation

Although it is beyond the scope and intent of this text to detail the principles and practices associated with pediatric and neonatal resuscitation, there are still some fundamental concepts that need to be covered regarding these special and challenging patient groups. Most important, you should be aware that cardiac arrest rarely occurs as a primary event in infants and children.

Trauma mechanisms notwithstanding, cardiac arrest in infants and children is almost always secondary to respiratory insufficiency. With infants, unless a congenital defect is present, you may be certain that a cardiac crisis will follow any serious unrecognized and/or untreated respiratory condition.

More often than not, in rare cases when a field delivery occurs, prompt and thorough suctioning of the newborn's airway, maintaining proper anatomic position, and being attentive for any of the signs of respiratory distress will prevent a cardiac catastrophe.

As a child grows, new variables come into play. Drowning, toxic ingestions of plants or medications, and trauma become increasingly likely as mechanisms to produce cardiac arrest. Probably the single most important point to be made about infants and children is their body's incredible ability to compensate for illness and injury. Because of this, they tend to compensate well until the "bottom falls out" and then crash hard. To help avoid such a catastrophe, do not delay transport of ill or injured children.

■ Vital Vocabulary

anoxia   An absence of oxygen in the tissues.

cardiotoxic   Describes any substance that is harmful or toxic to the heart.

cerebral embolism   Obstruction of a cerebral artery caused by a clot that was formed elsewhere in the body and traveled to the brain.

cerebral thrombosis   A clot in the brain that results in a blockage called a cerebral embolism.

cerebrovascular accident (CVA)   An interruption of blood flow to the brain that results in the loss of brain function; also called stroke or brain attack.

hemorrhagic stroke   One of the two main types of stroke; occurs as a result of bleeding inside the brain.

hypothermia   A condition in which the internal body temperature falls below 95°F (35°C), usually as a result of prolonged exposure to cool or freezing temperatures.

ischemic stroke   One of the two main types of stroke; occurs when blood flow to a particular part of the brain is cut off by a blockage (eg, a clot) inside a blood vessel.

reverse triage   Used in multiple-casualty lightning injuries; a method of managing a multiple casualty incident, in which the dead are treated first because they may be resuscitated with rescue breathing alone.

splash effect   A situation in which a single strike of lightning injures or kills multiple people.

tissue plasminogen activator (tPA)   A drug that improves neurologic outcomes if given to patients with ischemic stroke within 3 hours of symptom onset.

transient ischemic attack (TIA)   A disorder of the brain in which brain cells temporarily stop working because of insufficient oxygen, causing stroke-like symptoms that resolve completely within 24 hours of onset.

tricyclic antidepressant (TCA)   A class of drug designed to treat depression; when taken in overdose concentrations, these drugs become cardiotoxic.

■ Cases

1. You are summoned to a residence at 3:00 PM for a woman with a sudden onset of slurred speech, a drooping to the left side of her face, and a decreased ability to move the left side of her body. The patient's husband tells you that this started at approximately 2:30 PM. The patient is conscious yet confused. Her blood pressure is 144/90 mm Hg, heart rate is 76 beats/min, and respirations are 16 breaths/min and unlabored. You suspect that this patient has had a stroke.

   What are the two causes of this type of stroke? What is the main benefit of getting this patient to the hospital within 3 hours of the onset of her symptoms?

2. After loading the patient in case #1 into the ambulance and placing the husband in the front seat, you proceed to the hospital. En route, the patient's husband tells you that his wife has chronic atrial fibrillation.

   How might this cardiac rhythm have contributed to the patient's present condition?

3. You are dispatched to the scene of a major motor vehicle crash. On arrival, you find that there is one patient, a 24-year-old woman, who was ejected from her car after striking a tree at a high rate of speed. She is lying in a large pool of blood. You assess her and find that she is pulseless and apneic. You advise the police officer on scene to request ALS

support. You begin ventilations as your partner starts chest compressions. As you assess the effectiveness of your partner's compressions, you are unable to palpate a carotid pulse.

What would explain this? Would defibrillation be successful on this patient if she were in ventricular fibrillation?

4. After having been submerged in icy water for approximately 20 minutes, a young man is found to have no pulse or spontaneous respirations. An ALS ambulance is not available, and the closest hospital is 30 minutes away, so you initiate immediate transport and perform CPR en route. With the patient still showing no signs of life, you contact medical control and are ordered to continue CPR.

Why continue resuscitative efforts on this patient who has been in cardiac arrest for approximately 30 minutes?

5. After sticking a safety pin in an electrical socket, a small child was electrocuted. When you arrive, you find that the patient is unconscious with a pulse, but is not breathing.

By which mechanism did the electrical shock stop this child's breathing?

6. You are dispatched to an apartment complex where the police have just broken up a large party and discovered a young woman reporting severe chest pain. She admits to "snorting" cocaine that night. You transport her to the hospital, where she is diagnosed with an acute myocardial infarction.

In the absence of heart disease in this patient, what is the pathophysiology behind her heart attack?

CHAPTER 8

Legal Considerations

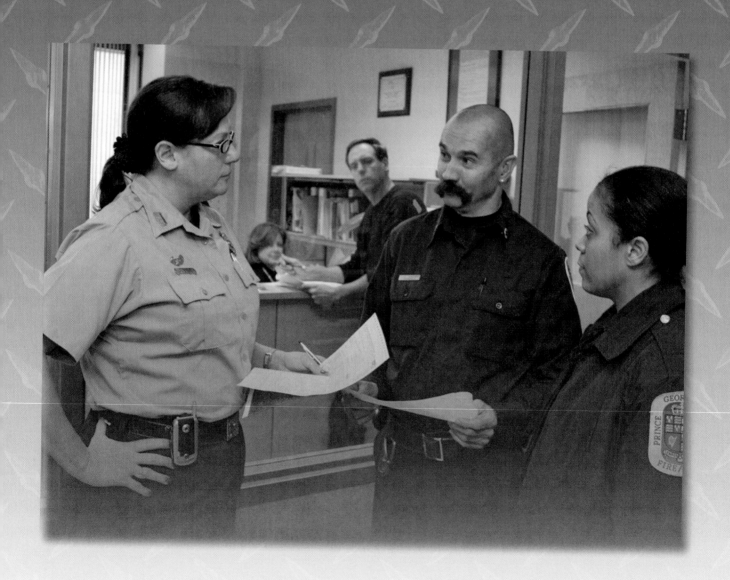

This chapter addresses a number of key legal aspects of emergency medical care. You will be warned about the potential threat of lawsuits relating to your treatment of cardiac patients or other patients who died or had another bad result, and how to protect yourself. You will learn about verbal or implied consent to treat, the extent of Good Samaritan laws, and advance directives or do not resuscitate orders. Giving depositions and other aspects of lawsuits are also discussed.

Unfortunately, bad patient outcomes are part of the practice of medicine. At times, despite every attempt to deliver the best patient care, your patient will "crash." When this happens, patient care interventions increase in intensity, with the goal being to avoid a catastrophic outcome, such as death.

With the varied range of possible patient outcomes comes an equally wide range of legal and moral quandaries. Although medical personnel would prefer that patient care not be complicated by legal or moral issues, it is. You need to be able to understand these issues and know how to act within the legal parameters established by federal laws or the statutes of your state and town.

In recent years, courts have shown a tendency to support the rights of competent, informed patients to make decisions regarding whether or not to have care provided. Additionally, should they choose to be treated, the extent of the treatment and care they will receive needs to be considered. In some cases, the wishes of the patient are in direct disagreement with the position taken by the physician in charge of the patient's care (**Figure 8-1**).

■ Obtaining Consent to Treat

From a legal and ethical perspective, patients have the right to make decisions regarding the medical care provided to them. Although a patient might not make the decision you would like them to make, that person is still entitled to make his or her own decision. In some cases, it may be a "bad" decision, but the courts have long ago recognized that patient autonomy simply gives the patient the right to decide, irrespective of whether it is good or bad. Whenever possible, medical care should be provided only after the patient has given consent. **Informed consent** is the most desirable mode in which decision making should occur. "Informed" means that the patient has a good grasp of the current medical situation and the treatment options. "Consent" represents the giving of permission as to which, if any, medical interventions will be performed. Thus, informed consent means that the patient understands the risks and benefits of the proposed plan of care as it relates to his or her particular situation, as well as the consequences that may result based on whatever choices are made by the patient.

Implied consent is a legal premise that comes into play when a patient is in an immediate life-threatening situation but, for whatever reason, is unable to state his or her wishes about the provision of emergency medical care. To ensure that appropriate care is not denied because of the patient's inability to communicate, the law relative to these situations works under the assumption that the patient most likely would wish to have the life threat addressed and go on living. That implication is the basis from which the concept of implied consent has evolved.

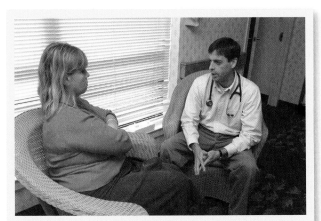

Figure 8-1 In some cases, the patient's wishes may be in direct disagreement with the physician's position.

■ Good Samaritan Laws

Good Samaritan laws and statutes exist nationwide and were passed to provide limited liability protection to people who, in good faith, stop to render care to an ill or injured person even though they had no legal "duty to act." These laws were focused on members of the lay public who may have little or no medical background as well as retired or "off-duty" medical professionals.

Laypersons or off-duty medical professionals have no duty to act. It is not their job, at least not at the moment when they come upon a person having a medical emergency. In order to receive the protection from liability that Good Samaritan laws and statutes provide, the person providing emergency care typically must have no duty to act and must receive no compensation for rendering care or providing transportation to the hospital. In regard to the quality of care rendered, many of these Good Samaritan laws and statutes use what is commonly referred to as the prudent man or reasonable man doctrine, which is what a reasonable and prudent person would have done for the patient if confronted with a similar situation. Good Samaritan laws and statutes, however, usually do not protect a person from acts of gross negligence, which is the intentional disregard of the need to use reasonable care, and as a result may cause a person grave injury or harm. In comparison, ordinary negligence is merely the failure to act or a simple mistake that causes harm to a patient. The difference between the two is the degree of indifference, with the lack of care in gross negligence considered to be willful or wanton (malicious) under the law.

■ Public Access Defibrillation Legislation

One of the fastest growing areas in emergency cardiac care is in the legislative efforts regarding public access to defibrillators. Many states have either passed or are in the process of passing legislation intended to do what Good Samaritan laws and statutes are intended to do, but in this case they are focused on defibrillation using automated external defibrillators (AEDs). In some cases, language about AEDs has been added to the existing Good Samaritan law/statute. As the availability of these technologic wonders increases, there are hopes that the legal protection these new AED/Good Samaritan laws and statutes will provide will encourage those in close proximity to the AED to provide care to the patient with sudden cardiac arrest.

Given the research already in existence regarding early defibrillation, many believe that shortening the time from cardiac arrest to defibrillation could be the most important advance in emergency cardiac care. This belief, coupled with the reliability, ease of operation, and low maintenance of AEDs, points toward a promising future in regard to reducing mortality and morbidity for patients with sudden cardiac arrest.

Many believe that in time, AEDs will become as common and readily available as fire extinguishers, especially in places where large groups of people congregate, such as malls, offices, schools, stadiums, and theaters. Widespread deployment of AEDs also may be of particular benefit to the BLS agencies serving those living in rural America, many of whom are 20 minutes or more away from ALS providers. In that particular setting, survival rates for out-of-hospital arrest are almost zero when defibrillation is unavailable.

■ Advance Directives

When they first appeared, advance directives (Figure 8-2) usually were drafted and signed with no input from the patient! Too often, patients were already mentally incapacitated and unable to make decisions about their care. Surrogate decision-makers, acting with a legal document called a durable power of attorney, made patient care and resuscitation decisions based on what they believed the patients would have wanted had they been capable of making the decision for themselves.

With the passing of time, the concept of advance directives has expanded, in some cases going so far as to legally support the decision or wishes voiced in conversations between the patient and family members, the physician, and sometimes even friends.

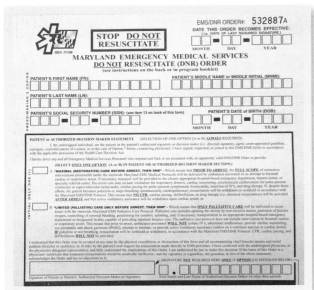

Figure 8-2 An advanced directive or DNR order is commonly used to identify a patient who does not want to be resuscitated.

TRAINING TIP

Have an in-service session for your squad on the various aspects of living wills, advance directives, DNRs, and durable powers of attorney as they apply in your state. You might want to include a lawyer or a hospital administrator in your discussions.

The laws and statutes relative to advance directives and **do not resuscitate orders (DNRs)** vary from state to state and go by a variety of names and titles.

Without question, written directives containing the specific wishes and desires of the patient, prepared when the patient is still mentally competent, remain the most desirable and most binding in the eyes of the court system.

Unfortunately, far too often EMS responds to an emergency scene of a cardiac arrest only to be told that an advance directive specific to a DNR has been signed. If this is true, the EMS provider may think, "Why was EMS called if the patient did not wish to be resuscitated?" Regardless, once on scene, the EMS team has a duty to act and care for the patient, unless legally relieved of that duty. A signed and valid advance directive with DNR instructions would serve to accomplish that.

However, unless an actual printed DNR document is present, the EMS team must provide care. Even if a family member or close friend says that such a document exists, the EMS team must have physical evidence in the form of the document itself. Verbal assurances of its existence from the family will not stand up in court. Whoever is making the claim that such a document exists has the burden of proof, meaning that person must produce the document. In case of doubt, contact online medical direction.

In a cardiac arrest situation, each minute that passes without a pulse or respirations increases the likelihood that the person cannot be resuscitated without significant neurologic deficit, if the person can be resuscitated at all. Members of the EMS team do not have the time to delay patient care in order to search for an alleged advance directive. The time spent doing so would compromise patient care, guaranteeing a poor outcome and probable death (nonresuscitation) of the patient. And, if no document is found or produced in a timely fashion, EMS would be negligent in the provision of care, or lack thereof. Therefore, if a valid advance directive cannot be produced immediately, initiate patient care activities. If the advance directive or DNR is located, a member of your team can contact medical control, relate what has transpired prior to the arrival of the document, and medical control can order that resuscitative efforts be terminated. In the case that a document is produced but is unsigned, altered, or appears suspicious for any reason, it is better to err on the side of the patient and provide care. When in doubt, run the code.

■ Lawsuits

Without question, it is much better and cheaper to avoid a lawsuit than it is to have to appear in court. Still, it is important for you to know that at some point during your career, you may be involved in a lawsuit. You may be called as a factual witness; you may be asked to serve as an expert witness in a matter in which you had no involvement; or you may be part of the team being sued. From a prevention standpoint, having a good bedside manner and people skills, including good communication skills, goes a long way in decreasing the probability that you or your team will be sued. "Please," "Thank you," "May I," and "I'm sorry" may be some of the most important words that any prehospital provider learns to use. When providers are rude and abrasive, they indirectly communicate a lack of concern for the patient and imply to others a lack of interest in providing quality patient care.

An indication that legal action may ensue may be when you are handed a subpoena for a deposition. Depositions are not always pleasant but should not be seen as the end of your career. Depositions are taken in countless cases that never go to trial. To allay some of the fear associated with being deposed, you need to understand that there are three main reasons depositions are taken during the discovery phase of a lawsuit (**Table 8-1**).

Having excellent documentation skills serves a dual purpose. It is one of the best ways to avoid legal hassles as well as to defend yourself should legal action take place. Many medical malpractice cases fall under the heading of what are termed "records cases," which means there is some docu-

Table 8-1   Reasons for Depositions
■ To discover the facts pertinent to the case.
■ To put the statements and positions of the witness on record so the other side can be prepared to respond to those positions at trial.
■ To evaluate the credibility of each witness.

mentary evidence that a breach of duty exists and substandard care was the result. This breach of duty can be documentation of a wrongful action having occurred, or there can be evidence of an act of omission.

The three most important things you can do to avoid a lawsuit are to provide quality patient care as specified by your service protocols and standing orders, be courteous and polite to your patient, and be sure that your patient care documentation is accurate and complete. In the unfortunate situation in which you are named in a lawsuit, these things will work in your defense and reduce the likelihood that the plaintiff will win.

■ Vital Vocabulary

advance directive Written documentation that specifies medical treatment for a competent patient should the patient become unable to make decisions; also called a living will.

do not resuscitate orders (DNRs) Written documentation giving permission to medical personnel not to attempt resuscitation in the event of cardiac arrest.

Good Samaritan laws Statutory provisions enacted by many states to protect citizens from liability for errors and omissions in giving good faith emergency medical care, unless there is wanton, gross, or willful negligence.

implied consent Type of consent in which a patient who is unable to give consent is given treatment under the legal assumption that he or she would want treatment.

informed consent Permission given by a competent patient for treatment after the potential risks, benefits, and alternatives to treatment have been explained.

■ Cases

1. You are assessing a man with a history of asthma who is very anxious. He has a prescribed inhaler and has taken two puffs without relief. You explain to him that his condition warrants transport to the hospital by ambulance. You further advise the patient that oxygen therapy and another puff from his inhaler are indicated. The patient accepts your suggested treatment and recommendation for transport to the hospital.

   Of what type of consent is this an example? How does this differ from implied consent?

2. While on your way home after a busy shift, you encounter a two-car motor vehicle crash in which one of the patients is complaining of severe neck pain and is still in the vehicle. After a brief assessment, you ask that patient to step out of the car and sit on the sidewalk until EMS arrives. The patient is later diagnosed with a cervical spine fracture.

   Having provided care to this patient while off duty, are you covered by the Good Samaritan act in this particular case? Why or why not?

3. You arrive at the home of an older woman who is found to be in cardiac arrest. As you are attaching the AED, the patient's husband tells you that his wife has a living will; however, he does not know its location. He demands that you take no resuscitative action on his wife.

   Because the husband has stated that a living will exists, should you attempt resuscitation on this particular patient? Would there be any legal ramifications if you were to honor the husband's wishes?

CHAPTER 9

Provider Care...Taking Care of You!

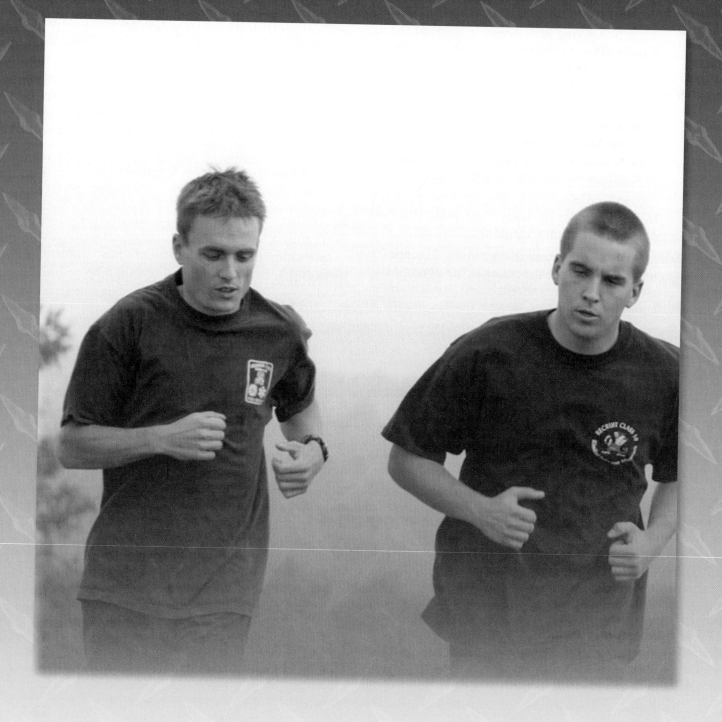

This chapter explores the high stress and attrition rates among EMS providers and gives you information on how to recognize when stress is affecting you or members of the EMS team. There are useful lists of the signs of short- and long-term stress responses, so you can know when you or a member of your team may need the support or help of a medical professional. Just as chest pain should not be ignored in one of your patients, the signs of stress need to be recognized and acted on to save the job or even the life of a team member—or yourself.

In the short time that EMS has been in existence, great strides have been made in improving patient care. In retrospect, however, it seems that the tremendous progress made might have come at a high price. Almost all efforts have focused on improving the training, education, and field performance of field providers. Unfortunately, little attention has been paid to the well-being of caregivers.

Provider attrition has been and remains a serious problem throughout the profession (**Figure 9-1**). Although the problem tends to be much larger for those who provide care through a volunteer service provider, full-time career EMS providers are not immune to the problem. Other than a few general surveys, there is a limited body of research available.

Despite this lack of research on this critical aspect of prehospital medicine, in recent years the well-being of the provider has finally begun to be addressed. In truth, all the technology, techniques, and therapeutic interventions mean little without healthy, well-adjusted care providers.

Prehospital medicine is frequently provided in dynamic and often unstable settings. Potential hazards and threats to the safety and well-being of caregivers are common. Recognizing and being able to control, remove, or work around these hazards are essential skills that must be mastered. Some of the hazards that you may encounter are shown in **Figure 9-2** and include the following:

- **Dangerous emergency scenes**—Emergencies can occur at any time or anywhere—highways, bar rooms, construction sites, and factories.
- **Inclement weather**—Unfavorable weather conditions may have caused or contributed to the emergency and may complicate patient care activities.
- **Hazardous materials**—Thousands of hazardous chemicals and other materials are transported and used regularly. Having a working knowledge of these materials and the additional resources that may be required to facilitate safe patient care are crucial.
- **Vehicles that are poorly maintained**—It is impossible to tell when and where the next patient may be found. Your emergency vehicle must be capable of providing safe transport for the EMS team and the patient.
- **Fire and explosion hazards**—Clandestine drug labs, especially those in the methamphetamine business, represent some of the most dangerous scenes in which to provide patient care. The precursor chemicals and the leftover waste products represent a laundry list of explosive, carcinogenic, and fire-starting or accelerant compounds. In addition, the people at the scene often are paranoid and well armed—a lethal situation for the unprepared provider.
- **People**—When emotions run high, judgment and common sense usually run low, making people arguably the most dangerous and difficult aspect of any emergency scene.

Aside from the challenges listed earlier, there are additional considerations for the provider who

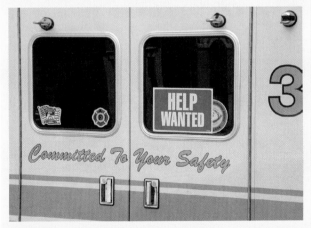

Figure 9-1 Provider attrition remains a serious problem throughout the EMS profession.

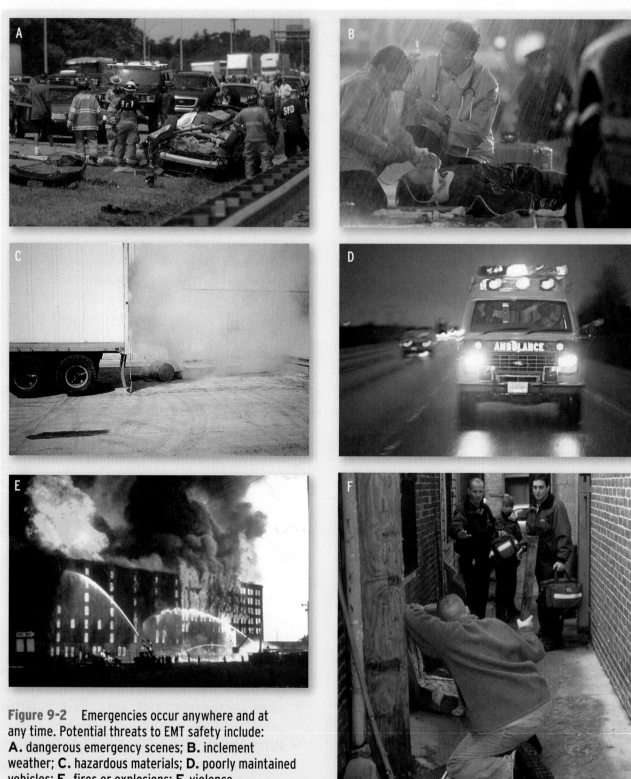

Figure 9-2 Emergencies occur anywhere and at any time. Potential threats to EMT safety include: **A.** dangerous emergency scenes; **B.** inclement weather; **C.** hazardous materials; **D.** poorly maintained vehicles; **E.** fires or explosions; **F.** violence.

wants to last longer than 6 months in EMS. These include the following:

- Managing stress
- Physical fitness
- Dealing with death and dying
- Poor nutritional habits
- Sleep deprivation
- Alcohol and substance abuse

Emotions, Medicine, and You

For patients and providers, unexpected illness or emergencies produce an adrenaline-fueled environment. Nowhere may those emotions run higher than when someone suddenly collapses from sudden cardiac arrest. If others are present and witness the collapse, whether they are family members, friends, or onlookers, the experience of watching someone die is overwhelming (**Figure 9-3**). When this occurs, EMS providers face one of the most daunting and challenging aspects of their job: bringing a dead patient back to life in front of family and friends. For providers and family members alike, emotions run high.

You need to remain calm, composed, and focused in order to provide the best care possible. You also have to keep the family and friends at the scene informed and be attentive to them because they are in need of care as well.

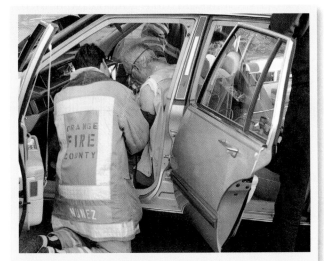

Figure 9-3 The experience of watching someone die is overwhelming for everyone, including EMS providers.

The Stress of EMS

The field of prehospital medicine may well be one of the most stressful of all the branches of medicine. Typically, a sudden, unexpected medical or traumatic event occurs, interrupting the daily routine of work or home life, prompting a call to 9-1-1. When compared with the clean, controlled medical environment of a hospital, prehospital medicine unfolds anywhere, anytime, and frequently under what only can be described as adverse circumstances. High levels of stress can be everywhere.

To be an effective prehospital care provider, you must understand the common causes of stress, how to recognize the warning signs and symptoms of stress overload, and what actions to take if you see these signs or symptoms in yourself or a coworker.

Realize that stress in and of itself is not a bad thing. In the right amounts, it can push your body and mind to rise to meet the challenge and bring you to even higher levels of performance. It is when stress becomes excessive and exceeds your usual coping skills and stress management mechanisms that it can render you overwhelmed and finally ineffective as a caregiver. There are two categories of warnings that your body will give when you are experiencing stress: the initial or immediate stress response, and the extended or delayed stress response (**Table 9-1**).

Both forms of excessive stress need to be addressed right away, because both affect your ability to make the key decisions required of a good EMT, and both are bad for your physical and emotional health. For example, if you try to ignore the initial stress response, either your own or that of a member of your team, it may result in loss of scene control and dangerously substandard patient care. This stress-induced inability to manage a call or to provide standard patient care may, in worst-case scenarios, result in a lawsuit, death of a patient, or the loss of public confidence in your EMS team.

Sadly, there are many emergency care providers who fail to accept that stress is a daily part of life in EMS. Long hours, poor diet, sleep deprivation, sleep pattern disruption, and uncooperative patients can combine to cause slow deterioration of a provider.

Table 9-1   Warning Signs of Stress

Warning Signs—Initial Stress Response

- Increased heart and respiratory rate
- Elevated blood pressure
- Dilated pupils
- Cool, sweaty skin
- Difficulty concentrating
- Inability to make decisions
- Sleep disturbances

Warning Signs—Extended Stress Response

- Personality changes (guilt, depression)
- Chronic fatigue
- Work problems (tardiness, coworker disputes, cynicism)
- Alcohol/drug abuse
- Change in appetite
- Decreased interest in sex

One disastrous event, such as a multiple-casualty incident or the death of a child, could leave you or one of your team members incapable of functioning normally. The suicide or accidental death of one of your team can be a life-changing event, and it may even cause you or another team member to consider leaving the profession altogether. The day-to-day stressors present in prehospital medicine can be subtle, taking their toll over a period of weeks, months, and even years. Do not be fooled into thinking that those extended time frames do not make chronic stress less damaging. They just make it harder to identify.

When stress levels overwhelm a provider's coping capabilities and mechanisms, it is important to recognize what is happening and get the provider the help he or she needs. Increasingly, private and municipal services are setting up employee assistance programs to help care for their providers. Although the informal support network that exists among providers is invaluable (**Figure 9-4**), there are times when professional intervention may be required to turn around a situation in hopes of salvaging a career.

In addition to the support and corrective interventions employee assistance programs can provide,

there are some simple changes that you can make or help others make right away.

- Match expectations with reality. If EMS providers think that they can or should save all of their patients, they are wrong. If they think that they will get 8 hours of uninterrupted sleep a night so that they are refreshed and ready to go to their part-time job, they are wrong again. When the expectations of a job do not match its reality, providers can become disgruntled, disillusioned, and disappointed quickly. Before you know it, one of the team is gone, adding to the attrition problem in EMS.
- Take time for yourself and have a life outside of EMS. Taking time off is essential to your well-being. Learn to say no to the endless opportunities for overtime shifts. Have friends, hobbies, and outside interests. Separate your work life from your life outside of work as much as possible. Make the commitment to a regular physical fitness or exercise program and stick with it. Try to eat healthy foods.
- Do not waste your career complaining about things you cannot change. Realize and accept that every industry has its problems, not just EMS. Each business has people who use and abuse its privileges. Patients are not always grateful. Understand that saving lives is not a daily event and that nonemergent medicine makes up most of what EMS is all about.

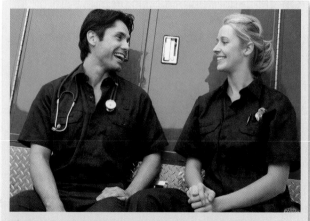

Figure 9-4   Informal support among providers is invaluable, but sometimes professional intervention may be required to help you or a coworker.

Recognize that life is not always fair and that bad things happen to nice people through no fault of your own.

Teamwork and EMS

Success in the field of EMS is invariably linked to the ability of the EMS providers and other responders to blend together quickly into a cohesive team. There may be no better example of that than in the realm of emergency cardiac care and advanced cardiac life support. Think about the following scenario: A customer in the checkout line at the local grocery store collapses from sudden cardiac arrest. Local first responders are on scene in minutes and administer CPR. An EMT squad with defibrillation capabilities from the neighboring community is another minute or two behind. They shock the patient twice into a perfusing rhythm and continue to assist respirations as they initiate transport. A few miles out of town, they rendezvous with a paramedic unit that assumes care and continues to stabilize the patient throughout the remaining 17 minutes of transport to the hospital. At the hospital, the paramedics provide a hand-off report, and the ED staff assumes care of the patient. The ED staff sends the patient to the catheterization lab, where an occluded coronary vessel is reopened. After a brief stay in the Coronary Care Unit, your patient is discharged and goes home to his family.

In this scenario, it is essential to recognize that no single aspect of a call is more important than any other. Each provider who cared for the patient was essential to the patient's successful outcome.

It is your skill and successful teamwork in EMS, and specifically in emergency cardiac care, that are the focus of this text and the associated coursework that it accompanies (**Figure 9-5**). The goal is to make you a better-educated, better-trained EMT who can make well-informed, positive contributions when working with ALS providers on cardiac patients. You are a key player in a team that increases the chance of a positive outcome for your patient.

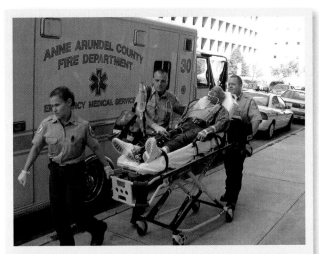

Figure 9-5 BLS and ALS teamwork improves the likelihood of a positive patient outcome.

EMS providers provide care to many thousands of patients with cardiac-related emergencies each year. This care needs to be as seamless as possible, with all providers doing their respective jobs to the best of their abilities, followed by providing accurate hand-off reports at each step. Positive, caring attitudes must be maintained from start to finish. Only one person truly suffers when the EMS system fails to perform as it should—the patient.

Again, the quality of the emergency cardiac care that is delivered directly depends on each provider involved in the continuum of patient care. This is why it is important to take care of yourself so that you can provide quick, decisive care to the best of your abilities.

Death and Dying

One of the most difficult aspects of EMS and specifically emergency cardiac care is dealing with poor outcomes, such as the death of a patient. One of the most important skills any medical provider can acquire is how to cope with and come to terms with the death of a patient. This is especially difficult for those in medicine who may see patients die each day. During the initial training of providers, many programs teach and reinforce the idea that if the provider does all the right things, in the right sequence and within appropriate time frames, there will be a positive outcome. However, outside the classroom setting that is not the case. Despite what you as the provider may learn from a patient regarding the emergency at hand, at best you probably know only a fraction of what has precipitated the cardiac crisis with which you are confronted.

It is essential for you to accept that even when all your responses and interventions are appropriate and timely, some of your patients will die because their hearts were already too damaged to respond to all the techniques, technology, and therapeutics that emergency cardiac care and advanced cardiac life support have to offer. Perhaps the facts will help you accept that death will occur. Historically, it is known that most patients (about 95%) who are found in cardiac arrest at an emergency scene will be past the point of resuscitation. You are there to do the best you can with every patient, so that there is a possibility of life for the patient. Do not take a patient's death as a personal failure. Your job is to provide each patient with 100% of your skill and decision-making ability. Do your best. When your best efforts do not keep the patient alive, remember that your best is all that you can do. Although 5% survival rates for cardiac arrest experienced out of a hospital are very discouraging, keep in mind that without EMS interventions, that survival rate would be 0%.

Anticipated Death

From a practical perspective, there are two categories of death: anticipated and acute. Each comes with its own circumstances and challenges.

In the case of anticipated death, a family member has been diagnosed with a terminal condition, and the choice has been made for the person to die at home (**Figure 9-6**). Historically, our culture has done little, if anything, to prepare family members and loved ones. The neat, sterile, stoic death seen on television, where someone utters a profound statement or two, then turns the head to the side and quietly slips into death, rarely, if ever, occurs. Often, a run of ventricular tachycardia or other cardiac dysrhythmia causes the patient's brain to become hypoxic. The patient collapses to the floor, in some cases experiencing a seizure as the brain

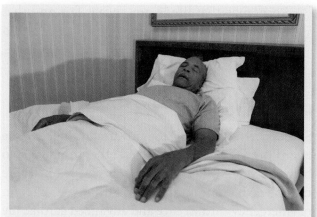

Figure 9-6   In the case of anticipated death, a family member has been diagnosed with a terminal condition, and the choice has been made for the person to die at home.

malfunctions from having inadequate oxygen available to meet its metabolic needs. Seizures can be quite violent and frightening for family members. When the patient goes into cardiac arrest, the skin assumes the bluish-gray tint of cyanosis. The plans to have a relative die a quiet, dignified death are disrupted by a much more harsh reality. In anticipated deaths, it is usually at this late stage that 9-1-1 is called. As the EMS provider arriving on the scene, you may know that it is too late or simply impossible to resuscitate the patient, but you face the task of dealing with a family frightened by the stark realities of death and unsure of what to do without a medical person in the home.

When you arrive at the scene in response to the call for assistance, you begin patient care. After you have begun efforts to resuscitate, someone in the home tells your team of the patient's terminal condition and his or her wish to die at home. A difficult situation confronts you at that point. Under the premise of implied consent, you have initiated care on an unconscious, unresponsive patient. The law does not give friends or family members the authority to stop the treatment. An appropriate question for you to ask of the family as one of your team continues attempts at resuscitation might be "What exactly would you like us to do?" If the person claims that a living will or advance directive has been signed, then they must produce a copy of a valid, signed document, as discussed in the chapter, *Legal Considerations*. If the person wants resuscitative efforts to cease, base station or physician contact is usually required.

Acute Death

While all life-ending events are extremely stressful, the shock of an acute, unexpected event is even more so. Again, resuscitation efforts must be promptly initiated to optimize survival chances for the patient (**Figure 9-7**). At the same time, several other actions need to occur.

In this situation, as you set up to begin resuscitation efforts, have a team member remove the family to another room or area away from the resuscitation efforts. Even a well-run resuscitation is disturbing to watch. Allowing distraught family members or friends to remain present only adds to their anxiety and yours. The additional pressure of having family members watch may distract members of the EMS team from the many tasks they need to perform quickly. Some studies, however, have shown that family members benefit from watching the resuscitation effort because it helps bring closure to the situation if the effort is unsuccessful.

If the choice has been made for the family to be sequestered, one of your team members will need to keep them informed periodically as to the status of the patient and of the resuscitation. All statements you or your team members make to the fam-

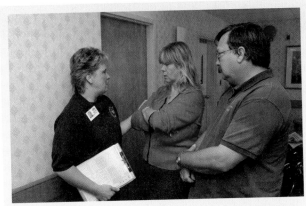

Figure 9-8 Sharing information at periodic intervals with family members or friends at the scene helps manage their stress.

ily should be made with compassion and be clear and informative. A comment such as "Well, it was going okay, but your wife kind of slipped through the cracks" only leaves family and friends confused and uncertain as to what you mean. It would be more appropriate to say "I'm sorry, we did everything we could, but your wife is dead."

In most cases, you and the other members of the EMS team will have a feel for how treatment is going based on the response or lack of response of the patient to your patient care interventions. A progression of statements shared with family members by one of your team at periodic intervals usually causes less stress than leaving them uninformed for 30 minutes and letting their anxiety build (**Figure 9-8**). An ongoing sharing of information in more manageable bits and pieces better prepares them for what is frequently going to happen—an unsuccessful resuscitation and the death of their loved one.

Grief and the Grieving Process

Grief is defined as deep sorrow or mental distress caused by loss, remorse, or affliction. As mentioned previously, coping with the death of another human being is a powerful, stressful event. Those present can react in a number of ways as the emotion of the experience starts to sink in. Unfortunately, one

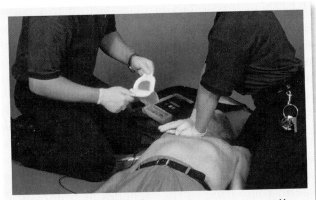

Figure 9-7 Resuscitation efforts must be promptly initiated to optimize survival chances for the patient.

Table 9-2	The Five Stages of Grieving

- Anger
- Denial
- Depression
- Bargaining
- Acceptance

of the most common responses is to verbally lash out in anger at the EMS team. When this occurs, it is essential to realize that while unpleasant and challenging to deal with, anger is a normal human response. Again, it is important for you not to take the verbal and angry attack as an attack on you personally. Because you know about stress responses, grief, and other emotions relating to death, you realize that you and your team are the most convenient targets for the frustrations of those present who have just lost a friend or loved one. This knowledge may help temper your own response or may help you keep another team member from losing control.

After an initial display of grief, those involved in the death will at some point in time need to accept what has happened. To get to that point, people often move through any or all of the various stages of grieving (**Table 9-2**).

Recognize also that grieving is a personal matter and varies from one person to another. One person may be angry and then in a few days or so quickly come to grips with the situation and realizes that a loved one is dead. Others may be in denial, ie, "He can't be dead!" As time passes, they may then move into bargaining, ie, "If they could only be here now, things would be different." This process may take weeks, months, or even years.

Still others may never overcome the grief, and over time their unresolved grieving may well become a life threat for the survivor. Think of a couple who was happily married for 50 years and then suddenly one of them dies. Three months later, the other mate dies. It is difficult to make a compelling argument that this is a coincidence.

Your goals when communicating and dealing with family members and friends about death should be as follows:

- Be honest and direct, yet compassionate.
- Be respectful of the seriousness of the situation.
- Use clear, easily understandable, and descriptive language.
- Treat the needs of the survivors.

■ Reaching Out to Others

One final difficult challenge on the matter of provider care include another difficult challenge and one that requires a proactive approach to truly be successful. It involves caring for each other.

There are laws and statutes mandating patient care, but there are no laws or statutes that require you to provide care to your EMS team. No laws require any EMS providers to stop what they are doing, turn around, and ask their partner any of the following questions:

- Why did you yell at and berate the last patient?
- Why have you smelled of alcohol at the start of the last two shifts?
- Why have you recently started sitting alone between calls?

This sample list barely touches on countless other examples that could and should be added if EMS professionals are committed to caring not only for their patients but for each other as well. You are in a profession where, at a moment's notice, multiple providers from multiple agencies or disciplines are asked to work together on behalf of one or more patients. It is easier to walk away from a coworker's problems than to walk back and offer your help and support. A holistic approach to caring for caregivers is needed if EMS providers are committed to the well-being of those who spend their time in the trenches of prehospital medicine.

■ Vital Vocabulary

grief A deep sorrow or mental distress caused by loss, remorse, or affliction.

■ Cases

1. You are a new EMT and are working your first shift. A call comes in for a 6-month-old child in full cardiac arrest. Despite your and your partner's best efforts, you are unsuccessful in resuscitating the child. When you return to the station, you tell your partner that you don't think you will be able to handle this line of work.

   What lifestyle adjustments must you make if you are to remain effective in the field of EMS? You feel that your heart is "beating a mile a minute." What is causing this uncomfortable feeling?

2. At the start of a shift, you receive a call for a patient with a minor injury. Your partner, an EMS veteran of 17 years, tells the patient in a rude tone of voice that he should not have called EMS for a minor injury. The patient, however, wishes to be transported to the hospital. When you complete the call and arrive back at the station, your partner lashes out at you for no apparent reason. As he is shouting in your face, you note the possible smell of alcohol on his breath.

   How can you best help your partner? What would happen if you were to ignore his behavior?

CHAPTER 10

Putting It All Together

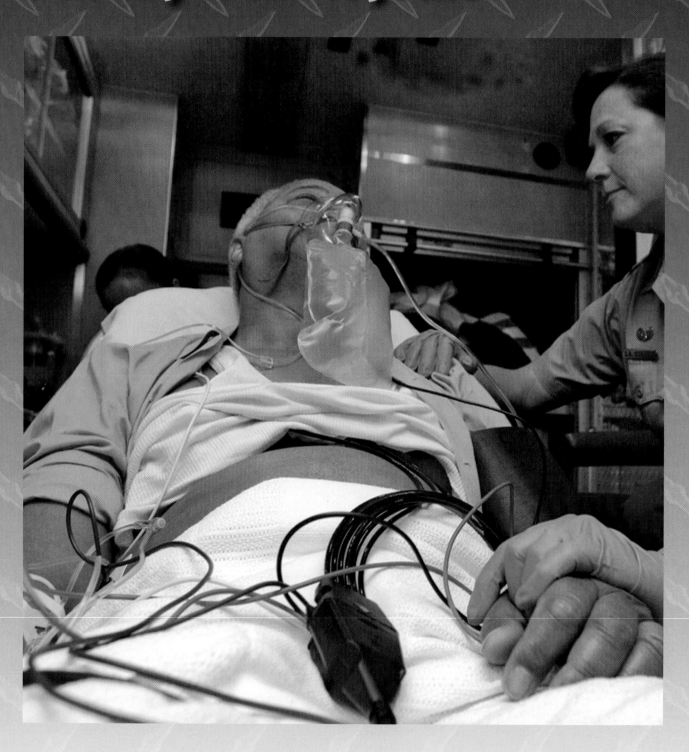

Thus far you have learned about the components of advanced cardiac life support (ACLS). This chapter helps you put it all together into the context of what you could do during one emergency ACLS call.

In ACLS, people, technical expertise, protocols, selected technology, and therapeutic interventions must be combined quickly and efficiently into a seamless cohesive effort. When all these parts are put together, the intent is to reduce patient mortality and morbidity.

Listed next are the nine key ingredients needed to provide optimal ACLS care.

1. Early Access to ALS

It is becoming increasingly common for BLS services to make arrangements with ALS services to respond either directly to the scene or to provide an ALS intercept. Both approaches focus on the same goal: delivering the same quality of prehospital care that people experience in the urban setting not only to the suburbs, but also into rural areas.

When ALS responds to the emergency scene in coordination with a BLS crew, it is termed a tiered or layered response. Your BLS team arrives first and does the primary patient assessment and work-up. On the basis of criteria predefined by local protocol, you then decide whether to request an ALS response. Your task is to perform the initial tier of emergency medicine: identify and correct life threats, call for ALS, keep the patient alive, and begin to stabilize the patient. Without this tier, there is no second tier. The second tier is the ALS team, which brings additional therapies to stabilize the patient further.

With an ALS intercept, your BLS crew also assesses and does the initial work-up on the patient. You or the dispatcher sets up the place where the ALS team will meet you. Your team provides the appropriate care interventions as you load the patient and initiate transport. The ALS unit goes to a preselected intercept site. When your BLS unit arrives, at least one and possibly two ALS providers join your BLS unit with their gear and transport continues, or depending on the condition of the patient, the patient may be moved to the ALS unit, which will continue

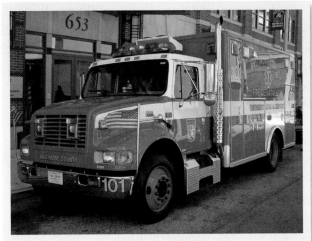

Figure 10-1   ALS care is built on BLS care.

the transport and allow the BLS unit to return to its community. The ALS team performs an assessment and provides ALS care en route to the hospital.

In either case, the real key to providing quality care is to be proactive in requesting ALS support. Your task as the first tier provider is to make a prompt, informed, and insightful patient assessment, and then make the call for ALS support.

Savvy BLS service providers usually adapt some of the decision making used in criteria-based emergency dispatching outlined by local protocol in deciding whether to request ALS. That, coupled with a solid primary assessment, gets ALS en route sooner, hopefully before the patient deteriorates or experiences cardiac arrest. Ideally, ALS and BLS combine their respective efforts and prevent the prehospital cardiac arrest from occurring. Just remember, by making a timely call to your ALS provider, you will have ALS support sooner. ALS care is built on BLS care (**Figure 10-1**). ALS interventions are too often ineffective if BLS interventions were not provided first or were not done effectively.

2. Chest Compressions

One of the most important contributions EMTs can make in emergency cardiac care and specifically in cardiac arrest management is to provide the most effective cardiopulmonary resuscitation (CPR) as possible.

It has been said that effective CPR produces at best a third of the cardiac output and perfusion that a healthy beating heart provides. Although a third of the normal output is not much, it is frightening to consider that with ineffective CPR, the output is lower.

Ideally, each compression should produce a palpable pulse, and the patient should begin to pink up or, in people with dark pigmented skin, become less cyanotic. Ventilations should be timely, in the right sequence, and of adequate depth to provide good oxygenation with the subsequent maintenance of carbon dioxide (CO_2) levels.

The relationship of CO_2 levels and the body's pH is very important in emergency medicine. As CO_2 levels rise, the body's pH falls, meaning the patient becomes increasingly acidotic (**Figure 10-2**). Coupled with the already poor metabolism that occurs during CPR and the many acidic waste products that ineffective metabolism produces, the patient's slide into acidity is rapid. Keep in mind that normal pH is 7.35 to 7.45, and that 6.9 is the lowest level of pH considered compatible with life.

Another key feature of CPR is that it provides the mechanism whereby the various cardiac drugs are delivered to the heart and the body. These drugs are ineffective if they are puddled in an arm just above the IV site instead of being pumped to the heart.

Finally, you can be especially helpful by knowing when to start and stop CPR without having to be reminded. Prior to a defibrillation attempt, CPR stops and everyone clears the patient. If the shock is ineffective and CPR is indicated again, it needs to occur promptly. If you are one of the EMTs performing CPR, make sure you know when to stop and when to resume CPR.

Mechanical CPR Devices

Several mechanical devices are available to assist emergency responders in delivering improved cardiac compressions when providing CPR, and while these mechanical devices have been available since the 1960s, a resurgence in interest occurred after the International Liaison Committee on Resuscitation CPR/ECC Guidelines were published in 2000. Not only did new types of devices become approved for use by health care institutions, but many of these devices were designed to be used in the prehospital environment. The three types of devices primarily used by EMS are piston type (popular brand names "Thumper" and "Life-Stat"), active decompression (brand name "LUCAS"), and load-distributing band (LDB; brand name "AutoPulse").

Piston Type

These devices typically consist of a board placed under the patient's back and shoulders to which an "arm" is attached holding a pneumatic piston over the patient's chest (**Figure 10-3**). The piston is lowered onto the patient's sternum in the same place where a rescuer would normally place the heel of his or her hand to perform manual cardiac compressions. When the device is turned on, the piston

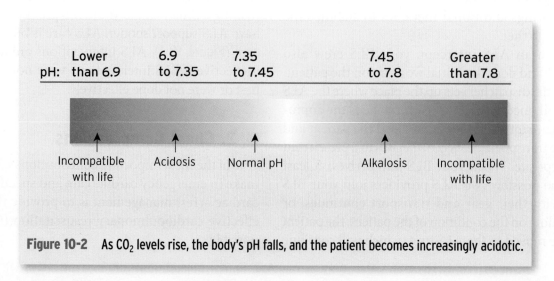

pH:	Lower than 6.9	6.9 to 7.35	7.35 to 7.45	7.45 to 7.8	Greater than 7.8
	Incompatible with life	Acidosis	Normal pH	Alkalosis	Incompatible with life

Figure 10-2 As CO_2 levels rise, the body's pH falls, and the patient becomes increasingly acidotic.

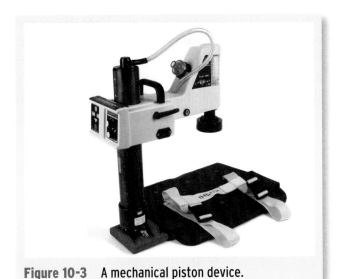

Figure 10-3 A mechanical piston device.

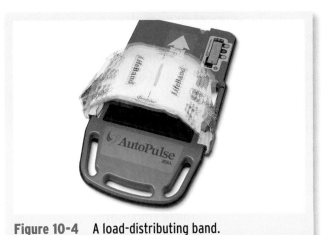

Figure 10-4 A load-distributing band.

cycles up and down in basically the same manner as a human rescuer. In addition to performing cardiac compressions, these devices often have a component that can perform ventilation as well, leaving the EMS team to concentrate on other aspects of resuscitation.

Active Decompression

Similar in many ways to the piston type, the Lund University Cardiac Arrest System (LUCAS) devices use a small back plate placed under the victim, with two arms holding a large piston "straddling" over the patient's sternum. A major design difference between the LUCAS and standard piston type devices is that the piston on the LUCAS device has a large silicone "toilet-plunger" style suction cup on the end. This suction cup is designed to provide not only active compression on the down-stroke, but also to "pull" the sternum back, providing active decompression on the up-stroke. The intention here is that the active decompression will lower pressures in the chest, allowing for greater blood return to the heart and improved cardiac output.

Load-Distributing Band

Using a completely different compression theory and design, the AutoPulse uses a small backboard to which is attached a wide band that surrounds the patient's chest (**Figure 10-4**). An electric motor alternately tightens and releases the band, squeezing the patient's entire chest, rather than directly compressing the sternum. The theory is that this circumferential compression provides greater cardiac perfusion pressures. An added benefit of this design is that the AutoPulse has a much smaller profile on the patient when operating and may allow for easier patient care and movement in environments where space is restricted.

Pros and Cons of Mechanical CPR Devices

Although there is conflicting evidence as to whether mechanical CPR devices deliver better compressions than manual CPR provided by an EMT or paramedic, these devices can often provide continuous compressions under circumstances where manual CPR would be difficult or impossible to continue, such as moving a patient down stairs or across difficult terrain.

The major negatives often associated with mechanical CPR devices are the trauma that is sometimes noted to the cardiac arrest patient and the cost of these devices.

Chest trauma is sometimes noted in situations where mechanical CPR devices are used; however, it is difficult to say that this trauma would not also have occurred from a human rescuer providing high-quality cardiac compressions. In addition, it is difficult to say that such trauma, often superficial soft-tissue injuries, would have any impact on patient outcome.

The investment in such devices is significant, not only for initial purchase, but also for provider education and ongoing maintenance. It remains hotly debated as to whether the potential benefits of using mechanical CPR devices are outweighed by the benefit that would be seen by an investment of the same amount of money and resources in public CPR and public access defibrillation campaigns.

■ 3. Cardiac Monitoring

Stay alert for the signs of impending disaster. One of the classic red flags is when the ventricles become irritable and begin to attempt to pace the heart. The beats that come from the ventricles early in the cardiac cycle are called **premature ventricular contractions (PVCs)** (**Figure 10-5**). These warning PVCs often indicate a slide into ventricular tachycardia (VT) or ventricular fibrillation (VF). With so many other patient care activities occurring, it is easy to miss a couple of PVCs here and there as they fly across the ECG screen. If you know what they are and what they look like, you will have a better chance of detecting them. Bring this to the attention of an ALS team member who may respond with treatment either directly, in patients who are either critical or particularly susceptible to VT, or indirectly, by working with you to address the underlying issues causing them.

False Signals

Be alert for sources of 60-cycle electrical interference, which include electric blankets and microwave ovens. If you can recognize 60-cycle electrical

interference on the screen and eliminate the source of the interference, you can instruct someone to locate the source and turn it off, keeping the monitor doing its proper task of monitoring the patient's electrical impulses (**Figure 10-6**). You may also have artifact from poor contact with an electrode. The solution is to press the electrode down firmly to make solid contact with the patient's chest or replace it, if necessary. Eliminating the artifact will help to provide a more clear, readable tracing.

This course is not intended to give you the capabilities to read the many cardiac rhythms most ALS providers can identify, but it gives you the fundamentals of the basic rhythms as well as some background on the most lethal rhythms that you are likely to encounter.

If the patient is in cardiac arrest, check for a pulse if you observe signs of return of spontaneous circulation (ROSC). If the patient is not in cardiac arrest, check for a pulse if there is any change in rhythm on the cardiac monitor (**Figure 10-7**). Minimize interruptions in chest compressions. The cardiac monitor only identifies whatever electrical activity is present. It does not in any way guarantee that what you are seeing is producing a pulse for your patient. That is up to you to determine!

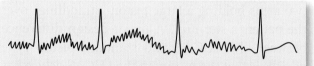

Figure 10-6   Interference by an electrical appliance in the room was the cause of this artifact. Turning off the machine caused the baseline to return to normal.

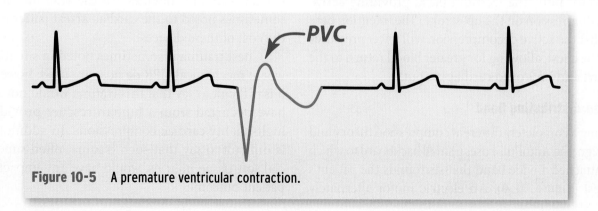

Figure 10-5   A premature ventricular contraction.

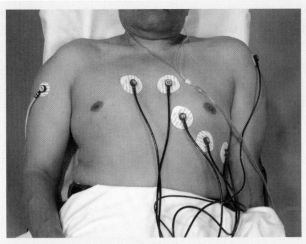

Figure 10-7 For a patient not in cardiac arrest, it is important to do pulse checks after any rhythm changes on the cardiac monitor.

TRAINING TIP

Learn how and where to apply electrodes for at least lead II and ideally for any lead configuration your ALS provider normally uses.

■ 4. Defibrillation

Rapid defibrillation relies on the prompt recognition of VF and VT. An extra set of eyes on the monitor increases the likelihood that it will be picked up as soon as it happens. Make sure to carefully watch the monitor.

In many systems, defibrillation is a skill that you may perform as an EMT. Make certain that you have practiced this skill until it is second nature, because this skill is often performed in one of the most stressful environments with distraught family members, friends, or bystanders looking on.

Remember that the person who is going to push the button to fire the defibrillator is ultimately responsible for the safe operation of the defibrillator. The components of safe defibrillation are listed in **Table 10-1**. Team members may be so focused on performing a skill that they do not hear the command to stand back. It is critical to clear the team verbally and visually before defibrillation.

Table 10-1 Steps to a Safe Defibrillation
1. Confirm that the patient is pulseless and in VF or pulseless VT.
2. Continue compressions while the defibrillator charges, thereby minimizing all interruptions to compressions.
3. Make absolutely certain that you are clear of any patient contact.
4. Confirm that other members of the rescue team are clear of any patient contact.
5. Defibrillate.
6. Immediately resume compressions.

In the event of a rhythm change from the shocked rhythm to what should now be a perfusing rhythm, make certain that there is a pulse check at the end of the next 2-minute CPR round. Again, it is essential to remember that the cardiac monitor only displays electrical activity within the heart. It does not guarantee a perfusing rhythm.

■ 5. Airway Control and Oxygen Therapy

Airway control and administration of oxygen are other areas in which you can assist the ACLS team. Airway control and provision of effective respiratory support in the form of oxygen therapy are cornerstones of good care for all patients, but especially cardiac patients.

Oxygen

If the patient's SpO_2 is <94%, oxygen should be administered to maintain oxygen levels above 94%.

Suction

It is important to have the suction unit ready. You know that nausea frequently accompanies heart attacks and if patients vomit, their airway may become blocked and require suctioning.

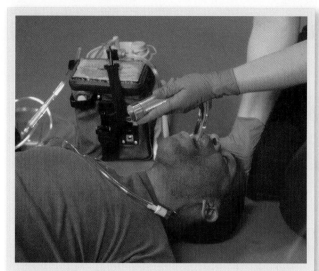

Figure 10-8 EMTs can help facilitate quick intubation.

Intubation

EMTs who do not perform intubation can help facilitate a quick intubation by performing any or all of the following functions to assist those who do (**Figure 10-8**):

- Preoxygenation of the patient
- Equipment selection and check
- Suction—is it ready to go?

Once the intubation is performed, tube placement is confirmed, and the tube has been secured in place, there is still key airway control work that you can do.

- Monitor and periodically reassess breath sounds.
- Ventilate the patient via the endotracheal tube with a bag-mask device with an oxygen reservoir.
- Monitor tube position for slippage/displacement.

■ 6. Intravenous Therapy

Starting an intravenous (IV) line on a scared, sweaty cardiac patient is not easy. It is a fine-motor skill that any good field medic will continue to polish throughout his or her career. A big part of that skill is making a wise choice of vein selection. Under

ideal circumstances, finding the right vein takes a moment or two, and on a very sick cardiac patient, it may take even longer.

You can help by using this time to find the right bag of IV fluid, hook up the administration set, and flush the tubing so that everything is all set and ready to go when the medic finds the vein to be cannulated. The following is a list of IV equipment with which you should become familiar (**Figure 10-9**):

- Constricting band
- Alcohol/chlorhexidine preparation
- IV fluid
- Administration set
- IV catheters (2)
- Tape
- 4 × 4s or 2 × 2s
- Occlusive dressing

Once the IV line has been started, you can help by picking up any sharps and disposing of them in the sharps container (**Figure 10-10**). This step is an important safety and standard precautions service. No one needs the stress of an accidental needle stick as a result of careless sharps handling.

During the course of the call, you will want to watch the IV bag and chamber to be certain that fluid continues to drip regularly into the drip chamber on the IV tubing, which will help to confirm that the IV line is still patent and running. If you see it stop dripping and/or you notice swelling at the IV site, this may indicate that the IV line has blown and is no longer functioning. You can alert the paramedic immediately so he or she can restart the IV line. In some cases, drugs that infiltrate into body tissue can be harmful, so let the paramedic know as soon as you notice that the IV line is not working properly.

TRAINING TIP

Learn where the various IV solutions are kept in the ALS rig and in the jump kits. Have an in-service session on how to properly set them up.

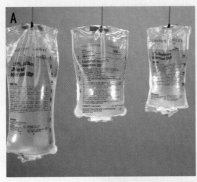
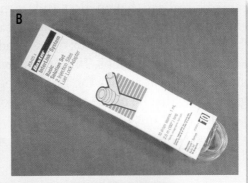
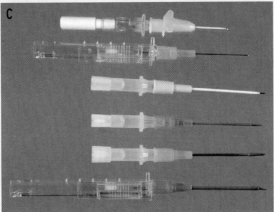

Figure 10-9 Some equipment used to start an IV line. **A.** IV fluid bags. **B.** Administration set. **C.** Catheters.

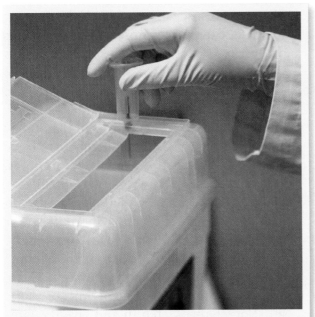

Figure 10-10 Once an IV line has been started, pick up any sharps and dispose of them in the sharps container.

■ 7. Drug Therapy

Without your BLS interventions, the patient may die, but BLS alone may not be enough to keep the patient from dying. Sick patients often need the benefits that the ALS team and pharmacology have to offer. Giving the right amount of the appropriate drug within the specified time takes a concentrated effort by the paramedic. In addition, paramedics must always consider the possible interactions that occur when cardiac drugs given in the field react with any drugs the patient may already be taking.

Your contributions in the drug administration process are to find and hand over quickly any medication the paramedic requests. You might think it makes more sense for the paramedic to keep the drug box close enough to simply reach in and take the drug he or she needs for the patient. Sometimes that is the case. However, the experienced paramedic realizes that an alert and oriented but frightened patient may become more alarmed when the patient sees the drug box open with its multiple drawers of medications. This may compound the magnitude of fear that the heart patient is feeling, thinking that he or she may die. Keeping the medication box out of the patient's sight helps keep the patient from becoming even more frightened.

■ 8. Documentation

As mentioned previously, one of the biggest differences between treatment in the field and treatment in the hospital is access to resources. Trying to accomplish all that needs to be done with two or three people in the field is far different than having eight or nine people available in the hospital.

The person in charge of the flow chart at a cardiac arrest has an essential job. If you are the person holding the chart, and you have accurate times as to when the various drugs were administered, procedures were performed, or defibrillations were delivered, you help link all the activities together. If the patient starts to deteriorate or does not progress as quickly or in the direction that is expected, the flow chart can serve as a quick and handy reference to review. For example, if epinephrine is supposed to be given every 3 to 5 minutes throughout the time that the resuscitation goes on, while you are writing you can also glance at your watch and let the medic know when it is time to administer the epinephrine again. Managing the chart or run report is another way that you can contribute to the provision of optimal ACLS care to your patients.

What if months or maybe even years after the call you find out that a lawsuit is being filed? An accurate run report is the single best defense tool at your disposal in case of a claim for damages.

■ 9. Scene Choreography

Another important role you can play is the person who provides the choreography of the emergency scene. While the dramatic events are unfolding, there are scores of small tasks that can make the call run more smoothly and effectively. As you know, every call is different and has many variables that must be addressed as they arise. This makes it impossible to provide you with a master list of what should be done on every call. However, here are some things for you to consider as you choreograph your next call.

- **Secure any possibly pesky pets.** Dogs in particular may try to protect the patient. It is best to secure pets in a bathroom or bedroom or anywhere they will be safe but still can be guaranteed to stay out of the way.
- **Shuttle equipment.** During a call, various pieces of equipment need to both come and go. This is where your logistical thinking comes in. Knowing which equipment to move out of the way and which equipment needs to stay close at hand is important. During treatment, this is even more important. You can keep the scene uncluttered by getting extra equipment out of the way. Field codes (cardiac arrests) are messy enough without having additional obstacles. Also, putting things back where they came from while the ALS team is at work means you are loaded and ready to go when the time comes to initiate patient transport.
- **Isolate family members and friends.** A cardiac arrest resuscitation, even one that is being well run, can be very upsetting to onlookers because resuscitation can look harsh to others with tubes going down airways, multiple IV sticks, defibrillation, and CPR taking place. If family members are calm and able to follow directions, it has been shown that it may be helpful in some situations for them to be allowed to watch the resuscitation efforts. This is especially true in situations involving pediatric patients. Otherwise, family and friends may gather together in a kitchen or other room so they do not have to witness the resuscitation. If that is the case, it is of equal importance not to forget that they are in there. Every few minutes, as time permits or as the situation changes, step in and give the family or friends a brief update. It may only take you a minute to do that, but the look on their

faces will tell you how much they appreciate anything you have to tell them and how hard it is to wait.

■ **Provide access and egress.** There needs to be a clear path both in and out of the scene for both people and equipment. Besides being able to get ALS personnel and equipment in and out, you will need to have room for a quick exit for the patient on the ambulance cot. Getting furniture out of the way by pushing it aside and clearing the floor of lamps, toys, or other small objects will keep care providers from tripping or falling, and hurting themselves or accidently pulling out the patient's IV line.

Being able to put all the individual pieces of the treatment plan together is essential if you are to provide quality care. There are many pieces—the patient, the BLS team and equipment, and the ALS team and equipment; each call is unique. ACLS is quite challenging. With all members of the EMS team, both ALS and BLS, working in harmony, a positive patient outcome is more likely to occur.

PREP KIT

■ Vital Vocabulary

premature ventricular contractions (PVCs) Ventricular activity that comes earlier than normal.

■ Cases

1. While you are performing CPR on a patient who has been in cardiac arrest for a period of approximately 5 minutes, your partner brings in the AED, analyzes the cardiac rhythm, and delivers a single shock as indicated.

   As you resume CPR, what signs would you expect to see if your chest compressions were effective? What are your goals in providing artificial ventilations?

2. During the course of managing a patient with a suspected acute myocardial infarction, you apply a low-flow nasal cannula because the patient is hypoxemic with an SpO_2 of 80%.

   What therapeutic effects does oxygen have on an evolving myocardial infarction?

3. You are assisting a paramedic in intubating an unconscious, apneic patient who has a palpable carotid pulse. The paramedic asks you to provide cricoid pressure.

   Of what benefit will this be to the paramedic? Of what benefit will it be to the patient?

4. Considering the skills that are within the EMT's scope of practice, how can you be most effective as a team member when assisting an ALS crew with each of the following techniques?

   a. Endotracheal intubation
   b. Intravenous therapy
   c. Medication administration
   d. Overall management of the scene

GLOSSARY

access port A sealed hub on an administration set designed for sterile access to the fluid.

acute myocardial infarction (AMI) Heart attack; death of heart muscle following obstruction of blood flow to it. Acute in this context means "new" or "happening right now."

adenosine A naturally occurring substance produced in the body; also used as a drug in cardiac medicine to slow automaticity and conduction through the middle of the heart. Primarily used to treat regular, narrow complex tachycardias.

administration set Tubing that connects to the IV bag access port and the catheter in order to deliver the IV fluid.

advance directive Written documentation that specifies medical treatment for a competent patient should the patient become unable to make decisions; also called a living will.

advanced cardiac life support (ACLS) The provision of emergency cardiac care using invasive techniques or technology.

ALS rendezvous or ALS intercept A model for patient care in which the BLS team receives the call and arranges for ALS providers to meet them at an agreed-on location, resulting in providing ACLS care to the patient as soon as possible.

alveoli The grape-like clusters of air sacs of the lungs in which the exchange of oxygen and carbon dioxide takes place.

amiodarone An anti-dysrhythmic drug given during sudden cardiac arrest when the heart does not respond to multiple shocks.

angina Transient (short-lived) chest discomfort caused by partial disruption of blood flow to the heart muscle.

anoxia An absence of oxygen in the tissues.

artifact Electrical interference that appears on the ECG that may mask or mimic the normal waveforms.

asystole A total absence of electrical activity on the ECG; also called flat line.

atropine A drug that increases the rate at which the heart paces itself by blocking parasympathetic stimulation to the sinoatrial (SA) node. This drug is used for patients with symptomatic bradycardias or other conduction problems.

automated external defibrillator (AED) A small computerized defibrillator that analyzes electrical signals from the heart to determine when ventricular fibrillation is taking place and then administers a shock to defibrillate the heart.

automated implantable cardiac defibrillator (AICD) A device inserted into a patient's chest designed to deliver an electrical shock if the heart experiences ventricular dysrhythmia.

cardiac continuum of care The collection of all of the different resources and services required to care for someone with heart disease.

cardiac pharmacology The study of drugs used in cardiac care and their therapeutic benefits, side effects, and administration.

cardiotoxic Describes any substance that is harmful or toxic to the heart.

cerebral embolism Obstruction of a cerebral artery caused by a clot that was formed elsewhere in the body and traveled to the brain.

cerebral thrombosis A clot in the brain that results in a blockage called a cerebral embolism.

cerebrovascular accident (CVA) An interruption of blood flow to the brain that results in the loss of brain function; also called stroke or brain attack.

coronary artery disease (CAD) Condition that results when atherosclerosis or arteriosclerosis is present in the arterial walls.

defibrillation The act of simultaneously depolarizing the entire heart muscle with an electrical shock in order to allow a normal rhythm to resume.

do not resuscitate orders (DNRs) Written documentation giving permission to medical personnel not to attempt resuscitation in the event of cardiac arrest.

dopamine An inotropic drug most commonly used to raise a patient's blood pressure in cardiogenic shock, usually administered by IV piggyback, and whose effects are dose-dependent.

drip chamber The area of the administration set where fluid accumulates so that the tubing remains filled with fluid.

drip set Another name for an administration set.

electrocardiogram (ECG) A tracing on graph paper that represents the electrical activity of the heart.

emergency cardiac care The principles of emergency medicine focused specifically on a patient with a cardiac-oriented problem(s).

endotracheal (ET) intubation Insertion of an endotracheal tube directly through the larynx between the vocal cords and into the trachea to maintain and protect an airway.

epinephrine A substance produced by the body (commonly called adrenaline); also a drug produced by pharmaceutical companies that increases the heart rate and blood pressure.

Good Samaritan laws Statutory provisions enacted by many states to protect citizens from liability for errors and omissions in giving good faith emergency medical care, unless there is wanton, gross, or willful negligence.

grief A deep sorrow or mental distress caused by loss, remorse, or affliction.

head tilt–chin lift maneuver A combination of two movements used to open the airway by tilting the forehead back and lifting the chin; used for nontrauma patients.

hemorrhagic stroke One of the two main types of stroke; occurs as a result of bleeding inside the brain.

hypothermia A condition in which the internal body temperature falls below 95°F (35°C), usually as a result of prolonged exposure to cool or freezing temperatures.

hypoxia A dangerous condition in which the body tissues and cells do not have enough oxygen.

implanted pacemaker A device that stimulates the heart to contract at a predetermined number of beats per minute.

implied consent Type of consent in which a patient who is unable to give consent is given treatment under the legal assumption that he or she would want treatment.

informed consent Permission given by a competent patient for treatment after the potential risks, benefits, and alternatives to treatment have been explained.

ischemic stroke One of the two main types of stroke; occurs when blood flow to a particular part of the brain is cut off by a blockage (eg, a clot) inside a blood vessel.

isotonic crystalloids The main type of fluid used in the prehospital setting for fluid replacement because of its ability to support blood pressure by remaining within the vascular compartment.

jaw-thrust maneuver Technique to open the airway by placing the fingers behind the angle of the jaw and bringing the jaw forward, which in turn pulls the tongue forward as well; used when a patient may have a cervical spine injury.

keep-the-vein-open (KVO) IV set-up A phrase that refers to the flow rate of a maintenance IV line established for prophylactic access, usually run in the 25- to 50-mL/h range.

lidocaine An anti-dysrhythmic drug used to raise the fibrillation threshold of the heart and prevent repeat episodes of ventricular fibrillation.

macrodrip set An administration set named for the large orifice between the piercing spike and the drip chamber. A macrodrip set allows for rapid fluid flow into the vascular system.

magnesium A naturally occurring electrolyte in the body; as a drug, it depresses the central nervous system, which may be useful in managing some cases of ventricular fibrillation in which the patient is resistant to conventional therapies.

microdrip set An administration set named for the small orifice between the piercing spike and the drip chamber. A microdrip set allows for carefully controlled fluid flow and is ideally suited for medication administration.

morphine An analgesic drug of choice when rapid anxiety and pain management are desired.

nitroglycerin Medication that increases cardiac blood flow by causing arteries to dilate; the EMT may be allowed to help the patient self-administer the medication.

oxygen A gas that cells need in order to metabolize glucose into energy.

peri-arrest period The period just before or after a full cardiac arrest when the patient's condition is very unstable and care must be taken to prevent progression or regression into a full cardiac arrest.

piercing spike The hard, sharpened plastic spike on the end of the administration set designed to pierce the sterile membrane of the IV bag.

premature ventricular contractions (PVCs) Ventricular activity that comes earlier than normal.

procainamide A drug similar in its actions to lidocaine, but that must be administered very slowly, thereby not making it the drug of first choice in cardiac medicine.

pulseless electrical activity (PEA) A condition where no pulse is felt on the patient despite having an organized rhythm on the ECG.

reverse triage Used in multiple-casualty lightning injuries; a method of managing a multiple-casualty incident, in which the dead are treated first because they may be resuscitated with rescue breathing alone.

sinoatrial (SA) node A collection of specialized electrical cells located high in the upper right corner of the right atrium that serve as the primary pacemaker of the heart; also called the sinus node.

splash effect A situation in which a single strike of lightning injures or kills multiple people.

sudden cardiac arrest A state in which the heart fails to generate an effective and detectable blood flow; pulses are not palpable in cardiac arrest even if electrical activity continues in the heart.

sympathetic nervous system The part of the autonomic nervous system responsible for defensive, compensatory responses; often called the fight-or-flight system.

synchronized cardioversion The act of simultaneously depolarizing the entire heart muscle with a timed electrical shock in order to restore a normal rhythm.

systems of care How EMS coordinates with other parts of the continuum of care and how all of the different parts actually work together—from EMS first responder to paramedic intercept to their coordination with the hospital and emergency department cardiac catheterization lab.

tiered response model Dispatch of both ALS and BLS to the same call. This may involve an ALS rendezvous or a direct response to the emergency scene.

tissue plasminogen activator (tPA) A drug that improves neurologic outcomes if given to patients with ischemic stroke within 3 hours of symptom onset.

torsades de pointes An undulating sinusoidal rhythm in which the axis of the QRS complexes changes from positive to negative and back in a haphazard fashion.

transient ischemic attack (TIA) A disorder of the brain in which brain cells temporarily stop working because of insufficient oxygen, causing stroke-like symptoms that resolve completely within 24 hours of onset.

tricyclic antidepressant (TCA) A class of drug designed to treat depression; when taken in overdose concentrations, these drugs become cardiotoxic.

unstable angina Angina that involves increasing pain and more frequent episodes that respond less and less to nitroglycerin or rest.

vasoconstrictive effect The narrowing of a blood vessel, especially veins and arterioles of the skin.

vasodilatory effect The widening of a blood vessel.

vasopressin A hormone that occurs naturally in the body, functioning primarily as an antidiuretic. It becomes a potent vasoconstrictor when given in large doses.

ventricular fibrillation (VF) A rhythm characterized by the absence of discernible waveforms on the ECG; a disorganized and chaotic appearing rhythm; the most common rhythm in sudden cardiac arrest.

ventricular tachycardia (VT) A rhythm characterized by wide complexes exceeding 120 beats/min on the ECG.

INDEX

PHOTO CREDITS

Chapter 1
Opener © Berta A. Daniels, 2010

Chapter 2
2-10 Courtesy of King Systems.

Chapter 3
3-3 © Tyler Olson/ShutterStock, Inc.; **3-4** Courtesy of Arbor Pharmaceuticals, Inc.

Chapter 4
4-2 © Tony Wear/ShutterStock, Inc.; **4-4–4-7** From Arrhythmia Recognition: The Art of Interpretation, courtesy of Tomas B. Garcia, MD.

Chapter 5
5-1 Adapted from Basic Life Support for Healthcare Providers, American Heart Association, 1997. p. 9-2.; **5-2A** The LIFEPAK 1000 Defibrillator (AED) courtesy of Physio-Control. Used with Permission of Physio-Control, Inc, and according to the Material Release Form provided by Physio-Control.

Chapter 6
Opener Courtesy of Rhonda Beck

Chapter 7
Opener © Keith D. Cullom; **7-2** Courtesy of Rhonda Beck; **7-3** © Jeff Thrower (WebThrower)/ShutterStock, Inc.; **7-5** © Darin Echelberger/ShutterStock, Inc.; **7-6** © Jamie Otto-coenen/Dreamstime.com; **7-T1** Data From: Centers for Disease Control and Prevention, Deaths and Mortality, http://www.cdc.gov/nchs/fastats/deaths.htm. Accessed 5/14/2012.

Chapter 9
9-2A © Mark C. Ide; **9-2B** © Bruce Ayres/Getty Images; **9-2E** Courtesy of University of Nevada, Reno Fire Science Academy; **9-3** © Mark C. Ide; **9-4** © Monkey Business/Thinkstock

Chapter 10
10-10 © Photodisc

Unless otherwise indicated, all photographs and illustrations are under copyright of Jones & Bartlett Learning, courtesy of Maryland Institute for Emergency Medical Services Systems, or have been provided by the American Academy of Orthopaedic Surgeons.

NOTES

NOTES

NOTES

NOTES

NOTES

NOTES